THE RADIOLOGY OF SKELETAL DISORDERS

Exercises in Diagnosis

Volume IV

Ronald O. Murray

M.B.E., M.D.(Cantab.), F.R.C.P.(Edin.), F.R.C.R.,
D.M.R.(Lond.), F.A.C.R.(Hon.)

Consultant Radiologist, Royal National Ortho-
paedic Hospital and Institute of Orthopaedics,
London, and Stanmore, Middlesex: Consultant
Radiologist, Lord Mayor Treloar Orthopaedic
Hospital, Alton, Hampshire; Heatherwood Hos-
pital, Ascot, Berkshire

Harold G. Jacobson

B.Sc., M.D.

Professor and Chairman, Department of Radi-
ology, Albert Einstein College of Medicine
(Montefiore Hospital and Medical Center), Bronx,
New York; Consultant in Radiology, Veterans
Administration Hospital, Bronx, New York;
Visiting Professor of Radiology, Institute of
Orthopaedics, University of London

SECOND EDITION

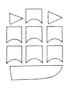

CHURCHILL LIVINGSTONE

EDINBURGH LONDON AND NEW YORK

1977

CHURCHILL LIVINGSTONE
Medical Division of Longman Group Limited

Distributed in the United States of America by
Longman Inc., 19 West 44th Street, New York,
N.Y. 10036 and by associated companies,
branches and representatives throughout the
world.

First Edition   1971
Reprinted   1972
Second Edition 1977
Reprinted   1979

ISBN 0 443 01267 9

Library of Congress Cataloging in Publication Data

Murray, Ronald O
   The radiology of skeletal disorders.

   Includes bibliographical references and index.
   1. Bones—Radiography. 2. Joints—Radiography.
3. Diagnosis, Differential. I. Jacobson, Harold G.,
joint author. II. Title. [DNLM: 1. Bone and bones—
Radiography. 2. Joints—Radiography. WE141 M983r]
RC930.5.M87 1976   616.7′1′07572 76-28430

Printed in Great Britain
by T. & A. Constable Ltd
Edinburgh, Scotland

APPENDIX

SUMMARIES OF SALIENT FEATURES

An Alphabetical List of Entities summarised in the Appendix
will be found at the end of this Volume.

TABLE IA. *Localised Congenital Anomalies of Importance*

	Spine and Thorax	Pelvis	Lower Limb	Upper Limb
Deficient bone formation (absence of bone)	*Hemivertebra*—organic scoliosis *Spina bifida*—minor forms common (20%) in lumbosacral area. Severe cases associated with meningocoeles and loss of pain sense. Anterior form: 'butterfly' vertebra. **22** *Absent sacrum*, partial or complete, **17** *Absent or hypoplastic odontoid process*—may cause pressure symptoms. May be due to infection or trauma. Not always congenital, **19** *Attachment of costoclavicular ligament (normal variant)*—defect inferior aspect medial end of clavicle representing attachment of costoclavicular ligament, **4**. Pseudarthrosis of first rib. May simulate un-united fracture, **6**.	*Aplastic sacral ala*—unilateral; Nagele pelvis bilateral; Robert pelvis. Deformity interferes with parturition	*Coxa vara*—(idiopathic of childhood)—varies from defect in femoral neck to complete absence of femur. Two forms: *congenital*—generally appears at or soon after birth; associated with other congenital anomalies; *acquired*—much more common and generally not recognised until ages two to six years. Bilateral involvement in one-third of cases. Pathogenesis undetermined. May result in premature degenerative joint disease, **24** *Bipartite patellae*. Defect always supra-lateral. Often bilateral, **4** *Patellar hypoplasia* with iliac horns, **50** *Recurrent dislocation patella*—patella dislocates laterally due to hypoplastic lateral femoral condyle, subjecting medial border of patella to avulsion strain, resulting in irregularity and fragmentation, **11**	*Radius and ulna*—club hand *Short 4th metacarpal* usually indicates generalised disorders such as pseudohypoparathyroidism and gonadal dysgenesis, **1188** *Erb's palsy*—humeral head and glenoid fossa are hypoplastic. Change reflects birth injury to brachial plexus; injury to phrenic nerve frequently associated, producing ipsilateral diaphragmatic paralysis, **12**
Increased bone formation (enlargement of bone or accessory bones)	*Cervical rib*, or associated fibrous band, may cause nerve pressure symptoms, usually asymptomatic, **11** *Accessory ossicle of cervical spinous process*—may simulate fracture *Sacralisation* of a transitional lumbo-sacral vertebra due to enlargement of one or both transverse processes. Predisposes to derangement of proximal intervertebral disc. Distal disc always rudimentary, **16**	*Iliac horns* (Fong's syndrome), often associated with hypoplasia of patellae and elbow epiphyses, **50** *Solitary enostosis*—represents cortical bone in medullary cavity. Such bone islands may grow and must not be considered osteoblastic metastases. May also involve appendicular skeleton, **6**	Bone enlargement by *arteriovenous malformations* (also upper limb), **1227** *Accessory epiphysis of medial malleolus*—often symmetrical. May simulate fracture, **4**. Other sites of appendicular skeleton may be involved	*Polydactyly*, may be part of chondroectodermal dysplasia, **154** *Macrodystrophia lipomatosa*—Bones of digits enlarged with large fatty masses in soft tissues, **13**. Differentiate from neurofibromatosis *Supracondylar humeral spur*—bony mass arising from anterior medial aspect of humeral shaft. Represents prominent attachment of pronator teres muscle. Fractures may occur, **4**
Failure of segmentation or congenital fusion	*Vertebral bodies*. Diminished A.P. diameter. Must differentiate from old inflammatory lesions. So-called 'block' vertebrae. Adjacent discs may undergo premature degenerative change, **17** *Klippel-Feil syndrome*. Multiple failure of segmentation of cervical vertebrae. Often associated with rib deformities and congenital elevation of scapula. (Sprengel's deformity), **20**	*Sacralisation* (see spine) of lowest lumbar vertebra, **16**	*Calcaneo-navicular* and *talo-calcaneal* bars may be responsible for painful spastic flat foot. Former shown in oblique view and may be incomplete due to fibrous ankylosis. Latter in axial view of heel on medial side of subtalar joint, **39**	*Carpal fusions*, usually unimportant, but again may be associated with chondroectodermal dysplasia *Radius and ulna*, preventing pronation and supination. Often overlooked for years

TABLE IA. *Localised Congenital Anomalies of Importance* (*contd.*)

	Spine and Thorax	Pelvis	Lower Limb	Upper Limb
Congenital dis-locations	*Hypoplasia of odontoid process* may cause atlanto-axial instability, **19**	*Congenital dislocation of hip.* Early detection and treatment can avoid subsequent disability. In neonates femoral head not ossified and femur displaced laterally from dysplastic acetabulum. Later radiological recognition easy. Minor forms also cause subsequent degenerative hip disease. Marked female predominance. Often bilateral, **8**	*Congenital vertical talus* due to dislocation of talo-navicular joint. Break in mid-tarsal joint with elevation of calcaneus and forefoot. Hence painful flat foot in young children, **31**	*Congenital dislocation of head of radius.* Always in a forward direction, often bilateral. Restricts elbow movements, **12**
Other localised deformities	*Various forms of scoliosis* (see page **990**) *Diastematomyelia.* Spinal canal split by bony or fibrous spur representing remnant of neurenteric canal. May be associated with *neurenteric cysts.* Spinal anomalies in cervico-dorsal area and cord symptoms, **22**	*Accessory sacro-illiac joints* said occasionally to be associated with low back pain, **18**	*Tibial bowing and pseud-arthrosis.* Often occurs in neurofibromatosis *Club foot:* Essential features—heel varus, equinus, pes cavus, and forefoot adduction, **31** Multiple localised anomalies with neurofibromatosis and arthrogryposis. Latter accompanied by marked muscular hypoplasia *Metatarsus varus adduction deformities.* Essential feature-adduction of forefoot and heel valgus, **30** *Pes planus.* Two types; simple and spastic (or rigid). Almost invariably bilateral. Flattening of longitudinal arch with valgus of heel in both simple and spastic varieties. In spastic form intratarsal coalition invariably present—most commonly talocalcaneal or calcaneo-navicular, **38** *Metatarsus primus varus with hallux valgus* (*'bunion'*). First metatarsal points medially and phalanges of first toe directed laterally, with subsequent enlargement of first metatarsal head. Development of bony prominence and bursal sac. Secondary degenerative changes common. Subluxations and dislocations of metatarsophalangeal joints of second and third toes may also occur in later stages. Counterpart of 'bunion' is 'bunionette' of fifth metatarsophalangeal joint, **41** *'Hammer toe'.* Mainly involves second toe but also fifth. Characterised by dorsiflexion of metatarsophalangeal joint, plantar flexion of proximal interphalangeal joint and extension of distal interphalangeal joint of affected toe. 'Mallet toe' is variety of 'hammer toe' in which distal interphalangeal joint remains straight and tip of toe impinges on ground, **42**	*Madelung deformity* of wrist due to impaired growth of distal end of radius and overgrowth of ulna. May complicate certain generalised dysplasias, **13**

TABLE IB. *Generalised Congenital Disorders*

A. DYSPLASIAS AND DYSOSTOSES*
(Listed in Alphabetical Order)

Disorder	Sex Pre-dominance	Dwarfism	Clinical Features	Abnormalities of Other Tissue Systems	Radiological Features	Remarks
Achondrogenesis, 142		Neonatal short-limbed dwarfs	Infants often stillborn or may die of respiratory failure in few hours or days. Limbs and trunk severely short. Abdomen distended and subcutaneous edema often present. Maternal hydramnios common		Deficient ossification lumbar vertebral bodies and innominate bones. Short horizontal ribs. Limb bones short with irregular flared metaphyses, particularly humeri. Bowing of limb bones not prominent feature	Often confused with thanatophoric dwarfism
Achondroplasia, 112	Females	Generalised but limbs especially shortened	Dwarfism, large head, kyphos. 'Trident' deformity of hands. Disc lesions in adults. Mentally normal. Classically circus dwarfs		Failure of cartilage proliferation causes shortening of limb bones, but normal metaphyseal width. Hence 'trumpet' appearance. Base of skull short and small foramen magnum may be associated with hydrocephalus. Vertebral body ossification reduced with 'bullet-nosed' deformities in thoraco-lumbar area. Narrowing of lower part of neural canal. 'Square' pelvis. Horizontal acetabula	Variants include 'pseudo-achondroplastic' form of Rubin. Differentiate from various MPS disorders. Arachnodactyly presents opposite features
Arachnodactyly (Marfan's disease) (hyper-chondroplasia, 1102		See under Table V—Metabolic and Endocrine Disorders				
Arthrogryposis (Amyoplasia congenita), 102			Contractures mainly in lower extremities, dislocation of hips, club feet, general weakness	Primary failure of muscle development. Skin webs	Diminished muscle mass of limbs, osteoporosis of long bones, flexion and extension contractures of joints, particularly lower extremities. Pathological fractures of osteoporotic long bones may occur. Other radiological features related to the many skeletal anomalies, e.g. club-foot, congenital dislocation of hip, vertical talus, calcaneovalgus deformities, carpal coalition	Abnormality of anterior horn cells of spinal cord has been reported pathologically. Most constant changes in skeletal muscles of limbs include diminution in size of muscle fibres and deposition of fat in fibrous tissue, resembling Volkmann's ischaemic contracture
Asphyxiating thoracic dysplasia of Jeune, 144		Mild dwarfism appendicular skeleton	Newborn thorax markedly narrowed. Respiratory motion primarily abdominal. Milder thoracic involvement may exist and may improve as infant gets older		Changes in thorax characteristic—short, horizontal ribs with flaring of lower ribs over upper abdomen producing bell-shaped thorax. Irregular, costochondral junctions. Marked narrowing of newborn thorax in transverse and AP axes. Abnormalities of innominate bones with cephalocaudal shortening. Reduction acetabular angle and retardation of ossification of triradiate cartilage producing trident configuration of pelvis. In appendicular skeleton long bones shorter and wider than normal with resultant mild dwarfism. Metaphyseal irregularity. Premature ossification of capital femoral epiphyses. Shortening of tubular bones, cone-shaped epiphyses of hands, feet and polydactyly	Is heritable. Transmitted in autosomal recessive fashion. May be confused with chondroectodermal dysplasia (Ellis-van Creveld syndrome). Mild forms may exist
Campomelic syndrome, 143		Neonatal short-limbed dwarfs	Anterior tibial and femoral bowing with skin dimpling. Macrocephaly, micrognathia, hypertelorism, cleft palate. Hypotonia and respiratory distress common		Marked anterior tibial and moderate femoral bowing. Short lower limb bones with hypoplastic fibulae. Secondary ossification centres of knees and primary centre of each talus small. Club-feet, dislocation of hips and knees. Lower extremities more severely involved, although bowing of upper limb bones and hypoplasia of scapulae may occur. Ischii show vertical inclination. Symphysis wide and iliac bones narrow with small wings and shallow acetabulae	Death generally before five months of age from respiratory disease

* See page 1961 for report of 'Committee on Nomenclature of Intrinsic Diseases of Bone' (Paris classification) prepared by C. Fauré, H. J. Kaufman, K. Kazlowski, L. O. Lauzer, J. Lefébver, P. Maroteaux, J. Sauvegrain, F. N. Silverman and J. Sfenger. This report includes a detailed classification of the skeletal dysplasias and dysostoses.

TABLE IB. *Generalised Congenital Disorders (contd.)*

A. DYSPLASIAS AND DYSOSTOSES (*contd*)
(Listed in Alphabetical Order)

Disorder	Sex Pre-dominance	Dwarfism	Clinical Features	Abnormalities of Other Tissue Systems	Radiological Features	Remarks
Chondroectodermal dysplasia (Ellis-van Creveld syndrome), 154		Short-limbed	Shortening of limbs most marked in distal segments. Polydactyly common. Nails of fingers and toes spoon-like and hypoplastic or even absent. Genital malformations—epispadias, hypospadias, hypoplastic external genitalia in quarter of cases Congenital heart lesions common—single atrium or atrial septal defect		Thickening and shortening of long bones, principally distally, with radius and tibia more often involved than humerus and femur. Excessive shortening of fibula. Dislocation of radial head because of shortening of ulna. Characteristic deformity of knees with widening of proximal end of tibial shaft and delayed development of tibial plateau. Bones of hands short with hypoplastic terminal phalanges and cone-shaped epiphyses. Polydactyly, carpal coalition, supernumerary carpal bones also present Pelvis shows trident configuration with bony spurs. Ribs horizontal. Skull and spine normal	Recognizable at birth and transmitted as autosomal recessive. High incidence in Amish population in Pennsylvania Must be distinguished from asphyxiating thoracic dysplasia of Jeune and rhizomelic achondroplasia Death in early infancy because of cardiac and respiratory complications in over a third of cases
Cleido-cranial dysplasia, 46		Rarely	Usually asymptomatic. Large head, narrow chest. Retarded dentition. Coxa vara may produce difficulties in ambulation. Cephalopelvic disproportion necessitating caesarian section in women not uncommon due to combination of large head of affected foetus and narrow birth canal of affected maternal pelvis		Defective ossification in (1) clavicles—usually lateral portion; (2) skull—Wormian bones, small sinuses; (3) symphysis pubis. Coxa vara and accessory epiphyses in hands and feet common. Short, hypoplastic distal phalanges of hand, elongated second metacarpals, pseudoepiphyses of metacarpal bases, 'cone' epiphyses and enlargement of ossification centres. Tendency for involvement of midline skeletal structures	Strong hereditary factor—transmitted autosomal dominant fashion. Defective ossification of membranous bone extensive in this condition, but bone of endochondral origin may also be affected
Diaphyseal aclasis (Multiple hereditary osteocartilaginous exostoses), 52		Localised limb shortening	Bony masses due to failure of modelling. Limb bone disparity. Nerve pressure symptoms occasionally		Cancellous exostoses arising near epiphyseal plate in long bones and growing towards centre of shaft in polypoid form. Exostoses often sessile in pelvis and, rarely, spinal neural arches. Disparity in length of limb bones common. Madelung's and reverse Madelung's deformity of wrist common	Strong hereditary factor in two-thirds of cases. May cause mechanical limitations of joint movement Incidence of malignant transformation probably less than 10%, although higher incidence reported. Innominate bones commonest site of malignant lesion
Diaphyseal dysplasia (Engelmann's disease), 88	Males		Pain in mid-shafts of long bones. Age usually 5-25 years on diagnosis. Hereditary factor now recognised, so that *Ribbing's disease*, with lesser manifestations of same type, may be regarded as a *forme fruste*		Fusiform thickening of cortex of midshafts of long bones. Progressive obliteration medullary cavity, but never affects ends of bones. Lesions usually symmetrical. Base of skull thickened	Infantile cortical hyperostosis affects different age group. Vitamin A intoxication should be considered in differential diagnosis
Diastrophic dwarfism—non-lethal form, 150		Short-limbed dwarfism	Manifested at birth. Micromelia, clubfeet, typical deformities of hands, abnormal external ears, restricted mobility of joints, progressive scoliosis, normal intelligence Dwarfism particularly severe. Thumbs hypermobile and abducted—'hitch-hiker's' position. Cleft palate in 25% of cases		Long bones broad and short with widened metaphyses, retardation of epiphyseal ossification. Invagination of ossification centres into distal ends of femora. Dislocation of one or more large joints—e.g. hips and elbows. Coxa vara common Most characteristic finding in hands—held in ulnar deviation. Short, wide tubular bones, underdevelopment of ovoid first metacarpal and abducted, proximally-positioned thumb. Carpal bones bizarre in appearance with supernumerary centres. Club-feet deformities characteristic. Metatarsals bowed medially and hypoplastic first metatarsal Spine normal at birth with subsequent development of severe and progressive scoliosis and kyphosis lumbar spine. Diminution interpedicular spaces of lumbar spine and maldevelopment of cervical spine with hypoplasia of odontoid	Genetic transmission by autosomal recessive mode Early death in infancy frequent because of abnormal softening of cartilaginous structure of trachea. Intelligence normal

TABLE IB. *Generalised Congenital Disorders (contd.)*

A. DYSPLASIAS AND DYSOSTOSES *(contd)*
(Listed in Alphabetical Order)

Disorder	Sex Pre-dominance	Dwarfism	Clinical Features	Abnormalities of Other Tissue Systems	Radiological Features	Remarks
Dyschondrosteosis, 182	Principally female	Mesomelic	Mesomelic shortening of extremities, bones of forearm and leg most severely involved. Limitation of motion elbow and wrist joints		Madelung's deformity characteristically present with radial shortening in relation to ulna. Distal radial epiphysis triangular in shape and underdevelopment of ulnar aspect. Bowing of radius laterally and dorsally and subluxation of distal end of ulna. Triangular configuration	Transmission by autosomal dominant mode. Pseudomadelung's deformity, resulting from trauma and infection, must be distinguished from true Madelung's deformity associated classically with this disorder
Dysplasia epiphysealis hemimelica (Tarso-epiphyseal aclasis), Trevor's disease, 73	Males predominately		Limitation of motion of joints associated with localised painless mass at affected site; pain infrequent. Secondary deformities such as genu valgum or genu valgus may develop. Usually observed in early childhood		Overgrowth usually of medial side of ossification centre with calcified mass simulating cartilage-capped exostosis. Affected bony centre may become massively hypertrophied, resulting in severe joint deformities. Lower limbs affected more commonly than upper	No hereditary factor known. Bony mass often does not increase relatively in size after age of five or six years, but new ossification centres may appear around affected growth centre, tending to fuse eventually into common mass which becomes part of epiphysis. Indistinguishably pathologically from true osteochondroma
Dysplasia epiphysealis multiplex, 72		Short limbed	Joint pain and stiffness, especially hips and knees. Hand deformities		Irregular ossification centres in hips, knees and ankles. Metaphyses frequently enlarged and cupped. Carpal and tarsal bones hypoplastic and short tubular bones of hands and feet tend to be shorter than normal	Must be distinguished from cretinism and Perthes' disease (hip). Although disorder tends to be self-limiting, premature degenerative joint changes particularly in hips, not uncommon
Dysplasia epiphysealis punctata—Conradi-Hünermann form, 148		Proportional or mesomelic	May be similar at birth to rhizomelic form, but tends to be milder. Intelligence normal		Many of the characteristics of rhizomelic form. Dwarfism of limb bones proportional or mesomelic and generally mild. Tends to be asymmetrical. Involvement, however, more widespread than in rhizomelic form	Transmitted in autosomal dominant fashion. Long survival the rule—often into adult life. Some infants manifest typical changes of this form but may not survive beyond infancy
Dysplasia epiphysealis punctata—rhizomelic form, 148		Proportional or mesomelic	Mental retardation, cataracts, cleft palate, club feet, congenital dislocation of hips. Thickening of skin, flexion contractures of extremities. Congenital heart lesions common		Multiple, discrete, calcified densities of varying size around joints, also in cartilages of neck, base of skull and ends of ribs, as well as posterior elements of vertebrae. Coronal clefts of vertebral bodies. Prominent symmetrical shortening of femur and humerus characteristic, with prominent metaphyses and thickening of diaphyses	Inherited in autosomal recessive manner. Infants usually die before age of one year. May be confused with Zellweger's cerebro-hepato-renal syndrome
Enchondromatosis (dyschondroplasia) (Ollier's disease), 104		Affected limbs short	Observed in early childhood. No hereditary background. Dwarfism common with disparity of growth between paired long bones frequent		Translucent columns of persistent cartilage (often calcifying), extend from epiphyseal plates into diaphyses of long bones. Proliferating lesions vary in size; may expand and thin cortex. Lesions in hands and feet tend to be aggressive. Soft tissue extensions not uncommon. Bilateral skeletal involvement with tendency to monomelic distribution. Chondrosarcoma a well recognised complication	Could be classified with bone tumours. When associated with soft tissue hemangiomata with calcified phleboliths, known as Maffucci's syndrome
Familial idiopathic acro-osteolysis (Hajdu-Cheney syndrome), 387			Generally apparent in childhood. Various developmental deformities of skeleton may be present, particularly hands, wrists, knees and elbows		Pseudoclubbing of fingers and toes with osteolysis of terminal and even more proximal phalanges. Genu varum or genu valgum, hypoplasia of proximal end of radius, subluxation of radial head, scaphocephalic skull configuration with wide sutures, persistent metopic suture, Wormian bones, poorly developed paranasal sinuses and basilar impression. Spine shows kyphoscoliosis. Severe osteoporosis often results in fractures at multiple sites, particularly in spine. Protrusio acetabuli and pelvic asymmetry common	Rare, bizarre entity of unknown etiology with multiple skeletal anomalies

TABLE IB. *Generalised Congenital Disorders (contd.)*

A. DYSPLASIAS AND DYSOSTOSES (*contd*)
(Listed in Alphabetical Order)

Disorder	Sex Pre-dominance	Dwarfism	Clinical Features	Abnormalities of Other Tissue Systems	Radiological Features	Remarks
Fibrodysplasia (myositis) ossificans progressiva, 1150			Localised, painful subcutaneous masses initially in muscles of cervical region, shoulders and upper arms. Progressive involvement of remaining musculature including back, extremities, abdominal wall and chest. Torticollis and thoracic kyphosis common. Increasing and ultimately total disability frequently, with remissions and exacerbations	Associated anomalies of skeleton common—digital anomalies in three-quarters of cases which may appear before ectopic ossification occurs	Two types of involvement: ectopic ossification of soft tissues and digital and other anomalies. Ectopic ossification generally not observed in early stages. Initial sites of involvement soft tissues around neck, shoulders and upper extremities with eventually large bone deposits in other skeletal muscle bundles. Ossified bridges adjacent to joints may result in bony ankylosis. Aggressive fusion of vertebral bodies reminiscent of ankylosing spondylitis common. Diminished growth of cervical vertebral bodies resembling Still's disease. Digital anomalies consist of microdactyly of first toe and thumb and phalangeal shortening of hands and feet. Synostosis may occur	Skeletal changes may appear before ectopic ossification. *Forme fruste* variants probably not uncommon
Homozygous achondroplasia, 142		Neonatal short-limbed dwarfs	Neonate shows disproportionate limb shortening more marked proximally than distally. Infants often sillborn. Head enlarged. Respiratory failure early		Large skull with short base and relatively small face. Short ribs with flared anterior ends. Hypoplastic vertebral bodies with diminution interpedicular distances. Short, square innominate bones with flattened acetabular roofs and small sciatic notches. Limb bones short with flared metaphyses and minimal bowing. Short, broad and widely spaced tubular bones of hands	Radiological features reminiscent of classical achondroplasia, but more severe
Larsen's syndrome, 182			Characterised by multiple dislocations of major joints with characteristic flattened facial appearance—prominent forehead, widely spaced eyes and depressed nasal bridge. Associated anomalies include club-feet, cleft palate, broad distal phalanges of thumb, scoliosis and infantile respiratory distress (abnormal tracheal cartilage)		Anterior dislocation tibiae and femora characteristic, with severe recurvatum deformity. Multiple subluxations and dislocations of major joints. Broad distal phalanges of fingers, mainly thumbs, and supernumerary carpal bones with abnormal appearance. Double ossification centres for each calcaneus typical. Abnormal segmentation cervical spine	Inheritance occurs in both dominant and recessive forms
Maffucci's syndrome (Enchondromatosis with hemangiomatosis), 1074		Inequality of limb length	Intelligence normal. Generally not before puberty. Multiple nodules particularly on digits and extremities. Unilateral tendency. Associated hemangiomata present in soft tissues. Pathological fractures not uncommon		Enchondromata and hemangiomata in soft tissues. Distinct predilection for hands and feet. Striking tendency for enchondromata to be very large and project into soft tissues. Growth disturbance of long bones common. No direct relationship between vascular abnormalities and enchondromata. Rarely, hemangioma may erode adjacent bone	Relatively high incidence of malignant transformation of enchondroma as in Ollier's disease. Hemangiomata cavernous in type with considerable phlebactasia; may contain both calcified and uncalcified thrombi (phleboliths)
Melorheostosis, 82			Pain, stiffness, limitation of motion of involved extremity. Various skeletal deformities common—flexion contractures of hips and knees, genu valgum, genu varus, valgus deformities of feet, dislocated patellae, discrepancy of limb length. Muscle atrophy frequent; skin may resemble scleroderma		Multiple areas of dense hyperostosis with tendency to linear, segmental distribution. Peripheral deposits on long bones generally. Usually monomelic; more common in lower limbs. Innominate bones, spine and thorax may be involved. Large bony masses may extend into major joints and soft tissues	Radiological diagnosis often established as incidental finding. Pattern of skeletal involvement and skin changes suggest widespread mesodermal disorder. Association with congenital A-V malformations

TABLE IB. *Generalised Congenital Disorders (contd.)*

A. DYSPLASIAS AND DYSOSTOSES (*contd*)
(Listed in Alphabetical Order)

Disorder	Sex Pre-dominance	Dwarfism	Clinical Features	Abnormalities of Other Tissue Systems	Radiological Features	Remarks
Mesomelic dwarfism, 164			Three types: 1. *Langer type*—characterised by mesomelic short-ening of limbs, hypoplasia of ulnae, fibulae and mand-ible, and normal trunk. Mental im-pairment. Trans-mission by autosom-al recessive mode. 2. *Nievergelt type*—recognisable at birth and characterised by severe mesomelic shortening and specific configura-tion of lower limb bones. Tibiae and fibulae show marked thickening in central portions. Club-foot often present. Transmitted in auto-somal dominant fashion. 3. *Lamy-Bienenfeld type*—characterised by shortening of radii, ulnae and tibiae, absent fibulae, and normal femora and humeri. Laxity of ligaments, especially in lower extremities. Trans-mitted as autosomal dominant trait		Shortening of limbs at birth, more marked in tibiae and radii. Modelling deform-ities with resultant widening of dia-physes. Mild to moderate bowing. Fibular and ulnar hypoplasia striking. In adult same proportions persist. Defective ossification distal end of ulna may result in ulnar deviation of hand	In addition to the forms described, dyschon-drosteosis is con-sidered a mild form, associated with Madelung's deform-ity of wrist
Metaphyseal chon-drodysplasia-type Jansen, 161		Short-limbed, severe	Intelligence normal or retarded, with clini-cal features de-scribed for McKusick and Schmid types exag-gerated in this less common form. Blood serum calcium often elevated		Epiphyseal plates grossly widened al-though ossification centres normal. Metaphyses grossly expanded, irregular and fragmented, with irregular lucen-cies representing unossified cartilage extending into diaphyses. Both long and short tubular bones affected with distribution symmetrical. Skeletal changes closely resemble rickets in neonates and infancy.	Occurrence tends to be sporadic Other less common forms of MCD with lesser degrees of de-formity exist. Wide spectrum of changes
Metaphyseal chon-drodysplasia —type McKusick (cartilage-hair-hypoplasia), 160		Short-limbed and severe	Sparse, brittle head and body hair with deficient pigmenta-tion. Normal intel-ligence. Short trunk. Hands and feet relatively small. Fingers short and hyperextens-ible. Pectus carinatum with prominent thoracic costochondral junc-tions and Harrison's grooves		Shortening of long bones with normal width. Cupped and widened meta-physes and lucent defects. Ossification centers flattened Hands relatively small. Middle phalanges most affected. Distal phalanges narrow throughout child-hood, subsequently becoming triangu-lar and bullet-shaped. Feet show simi-lar but less severe changes Widened costochondral junctions with cystic lucencies. Pectus carinatum. Skull normal and spine abnormalities minimal with relative decrease in sagit-tal and coronal dimensions of vertebral bodies. Lumbar lordosis Pelvic changes variable and include out-ward flaring of iliac bones and narrow-ing of pelvic outlet	Initially described in Amish in United States. Transmitted in autosomal reces-sive mode Skeletal abnormalities tend to diminish in severity with ageing
Metaphyseal chon-drodysplasia —type Schmid, 158			Short stature with shor-tened and bowed long bones, lumbar lordosis and wad-dling gait		Changes in long bones reminiscent of vitamin D refractory rickets; blood chemical studies normal. Epiphyseal growth plates widened with metaphyses irregular, widened and cupped. More marked lower limbs. Coxa vara and genu varum. Mild involvement of hands and wrists	Transmitted in auto-somal dominant fashion. Common-est form of meta-physeal chondro-dysplasia group
Metaphyseal dys-plasia (Pyle's dis-ease), 75		Often tall	Often asymptomatic. Bulbous enlarge-ment ends of long bones. Genu val-gum. Facies show coarse features		Major long bones mainly affected, with splaying of proximal and distal ends and relative constriction central portions of shafts. Also tubular bones of hands, medial ends of clavicles, sternal ends of ribs and innominate bones. Cortices of widened bone ends thinned	Skull and facial bones thickened and dense. Spine shows flattened vertebral bodies with central densities

TABLE IB. *Generalised Congenital Disorders (contd.)*

A. DYSPLASIAS AND DYSOSTOSES (*contd*)
(Listed in Alphabetical Order)

Disorder	Sex Pre-dominance	Dwarfism	Clinical Features	Abnormalities of Other Tissue Systems	Radiological Features	Remarks
Metatropic dwarfism, 166		Short-limbed	Limbs short and trunk disproportionately elongated. Progressive reversal ratio of length of trunk to extremities with progressive kyphoscoliosis. Skull and facies normal. Major joints—e.g. knees—enlarged with decreased mobility. Longitudinal, caudal, double skin fold overlies coccygeal region Neonate thorax long and narrowed with sternal protrusion. In older child chin may rest on sternum. Persistent respiratory distress. Hypoplasia of odontoid process and consequently atlanto-axial instability		In neonate platyspondyly with very wide intervertebral spaces. Wedge or 'keel-shaped' vertebral bodies Pelvis characteristic with short and squared iliac bones, irregular acetabula and narrowed greater sciatic notches Short to widened ribs resulting in cylindrically narrowed, elongated thorax. Pectus carinatum common Long bones short with exaggerated metaphyseal widening or flaring. Prominent articular cartilages produce wide separation of major joint spaces. Delay in ossification of flattened and irregular epiphyses. Phalanges of hands shortened with widened ends—'hour-glass' configuration	Must be distinguished from achondroplasia and mucopolysaccharidoses
Neurofibromatosis, 58		Caused by scoliosis	Cutaneous manifestations—café-au-lait patches, molluscum fibrosum. Nerve sheath tumours. Scoliosis. Various congenital deformities	Skin changes—pigmentation and molluscum fibrosum. Optic nerve gliomata not uncommon. Increased incidence of intracranial meningioma. Neurofibromata in gastrointestinal tract and other structures Occlusive disease of renal arteries or aorta; aneurysms renal arteries. Associated osteomalacia may occur	Skeletal features include: (1) disturbances of growth usually hyperplastic (may be hypoplastic); (2) abnormalities of bone texture—distinctive, streaky, medullary pattern particularly in long bones; (3) pseudoarthrosis of long bone frequent—most common in tibia, although may occur in any long bone; (4) erosions of skeleton caused by pressure of neurofibroma, although actual tumour not always present; (5) *skull*—asymmetry and failure of development of sphenoid bone and posterior wall of orbit. Radiolucent defect adjacent to lambdoidal suture rarely; (6) *spine*—kyphoscoliosis or scoliosis in approximately half the cases—short-curve in type. Intervertebral foramina often enlarged. Posterior concavities ('scalloping') reflect actual expansion of neural canal by internal meningocoeles or arachnoid cysts. Lateral meningocoeles may occur; (7) *thorax*—deformed with attenuated ribs, particularly in upper portion of thorax—'twisted' ribs reminiscent of osteogenesis imperfecta	Malignant neoplasia a complication in approximately 10% of cases. Associated congenital anomalies such as vertebral fusion, spina bifida, and congenital hip dislocation not uncommon
Osteogenesis imperfecta, 94		May be generalised	Blue sclerae, deafness, multiple fractures with secondary abnormalities. Three forms recognised: infantile form; intermediate form appearing in early childhood; tarda form		In infantile and intermediate forms skeletal involvement widespread with considerable cortical thinning and diffuse demineralisation. Deformities of lower limb bones. Ribs attenuated. Wormian bones and basilar impression common Fractures at multiple sites hallmark of disorder. Compression fractures of vertebral bodies also observed, with biconcave configuration ('fish vertebra') Long bones may have appearance of being 'thick'—from innumerable fractures Tarda form relatively uncommon, with diagnosis often made incidentally in later years	Hereditary generalised mesenchymal disorder transmitted usually as dominant gene Pseudotumours due to callus formation as result of fractures not uncommon and cystic lesions may be observed Frequent finding—ossification of intraosseous membrane between radius and ulna
Osteopathia striata, 86		None			Vertical bands of density, most prominent in metaphyseal areas of major long bones, but sometimes in innominate bones and vertebral bodies	Usually incidental finding but may be associated with other sclerosing lesions
Osteopetrosis (marble bones, Albers-Schönberg disease), 80			Failure to thrive, premature senile appearance of facies, deafness, optic atrophy, hydrocephalus, nystagmus, severe dental caries, central nervous system findings associated with subarachnoid hemorrhage due to thrombocytopenia and severe anemia. Hepatosplenomegaly and lymphadenopathy common Benign and malignant forms recognised, with most infants of latter form stillborn or dying shortly after birth		Disseminated overall increase in bone density, with obliteration of normal trabecular pattern. 'Bone within a bone' appearance. Modeling of long bones impaired, resulting in expansion of ends of long bones. Alternating rings of increased and diminished density in innominate bones, suggesting heavy metal intoxication. 'Sandwich' vertebrae in spine. Skull changes variable, consisting of increased density of basal segments. Prognathism may develop. Bones brittle and fracture easily	Disorder probably due to failure of osteoclastic resorption. Survival beyond middle life uncommon. Death often because of recurrent infection, massive haemorrhage, terminal leukemia. Benign form—dominant gene, malignant form—autosomal recessive gene

TABLE IB. *Generalised Congenital Disorders* (*contd.*)

A. DYSPLASIAS AND DYSOSTOSES (*contd*)
(Listed in Alphabetical Order)

Disorder	Sex Pre-dominance	Dwarfism	Clinical Features	Abnormalities of Other Tissue Systems	Radiological Features	Remarks
Osteopoikilosis, 84	Males		None. Often hereditary		Multiple islands of increased density in cancellous bone, oval or round and varying from 2 to 10 mm in diameter. Epiphyseal and metaphyseal areas most affected especially wrist, ankle and pelvis	Always an incidental finding
Phocomelia, 187			May affect one or more limbs symmetrically or asymmetrically. Several forms show familial transmission as isolated anomalies. Many anomalies may occur	May have multiple congenital anomalies	Three basic types: (1) complete phocomelia—absence of long bones so that hand or foot articulate directly with trunk; (2) proximal phocomelia—humerus and femur absent; (3) distal phocomelia—bones of forearm or leg lacking. In last 2 types remaining long bones often hypoplastic	Thalidomide ingested during pregnancy has resulted in birth of number of infants of complete phocomelic type. Femoral hypoplasia or proximal phocomelia, with accompanying sacral and coccygeal agenesis as result of maternal diabetes, may occur
Progeria (Hutchinson-Gilford's Syndrome), 186	None	Generalised	Affected infants normal at birth. Later retardation of growth. Skin thinned and atrophic. Head proportionately large in comparison with small body. Typical facies. Teeth and nails abnormal. Body small with thin extremities and prominent, incompletely extended major joints. Intelligence normal or above normal. Evidence of premature aging		Cranial vault thin. Wormian bones, late closure fontanelles and disproportionately small and narrow maxilla and mandible common. Obtuse angle of mandible. Thorax narrow with slender ribs. Progressive resorption and fibrous replacement outer portions of clavicles is hallmark. Evidence of arteriosclerotic heart disease on chest films. Generalised osteoporosis prominent. Long bones shortened and gracile. Coxa valga characteristic. Valgus of humeral head. Osteolysis distal phalanges of hands—occasionally. Vascular calcifications soft tissues common	Early death from complications of atherosclerosis. Cockayne's syndrome superficially resembles progeria but children with Cockayne's syndrome show mental retardation, retinal atrophy, deafness and family history, which permits differentiation
Pyknodysostosis, 1180			Dwarfism, widened hands and feet, dystrophic nails, characteristic facies (beaked nose, receding jaw), mental retardation		Bone defects comparable to cleido-cranial dysplasia, of which it is likely to be a variant, with generalised osteosclerosis. Wide skull sutures. Small facial bones. Aplasia of terminal phalanges	Strong, hereditary factor. Occasional additional abnormalities such as cleft palate, suggest the entity to be a dysostosis
Spondyloepiphyseal Dysplasia—congenita type, 172		short-limbed	Newborn infants short. Facies flattened and hypoplastic with cleft palate. Disproportionate dwarfism with spine and hips considerably more involved than extremities. Short neck with pectus carinatum and lumbar lordosis. Muscular weakness with abnormal waddling gait. Deafness and serious ocular abnormalities with retinal detachment		Newborn infant shows slight shortening of extremities. Multiple accessory epiphyses in hands and feet. Severe coxa valga and genu varum. Ossification centres of vertebral bodies incompletely fused with platyspondyly. Iliac bones broadened at bases with deficient ossification of pubis as well as calcaneus, talus and epiphyses of knees. Ossification abnormalities most severe in spine, pelvis and hips. Thoracic kyphosis and lumbar lordosis exaggerated during childhood. Odontoid hypoplasia apparent. Vertebral flattening and irregularity persistent into adult life, with narrowing of disc spaces resulting in shortening of trunk. During infancy and childhood iliac bones appear vertically short with wide bases and flattened acetabular roofs. Severe coxa vara and genu valgum	May be transmitted in autosomal dominant fashion, although most cases appear sporadically
Spondyloepiphyseal Dysplasia—pseudoachondroplastic type, 172		Short-limbed	Muscular weakness, late onset of walking, abnormal waddling or stiff-legged gait, dwarfism, spinal scoliosis and varying orthopaedic abnormalities, particularly hips and knees		Long bones more affected than spine, being short and flared with irregularly fragmented metaphyses and small irregular ossification centres. Bowing of long bones and uneven growth of epiphyses and metaphyses may result in genu varum and genu recurvatum. Tubular bones of hands may be shortened. Iliac wings flared and acetabular roofs flattened. Severe coxa vara common with subluxation and dislocation femoral heads. In spine, scoliosis, anterior tongue-like protrusions and platyspondyly in later years. Odontoid hypoplasia uncommon	This type sometimes divided into four sub-groups based on four separate kindreds. Transmission principally in autosomal dominant fashion

TABLE IB. *Generalised Congenital Disorders (contd.)*

A. DYSPLASIAS AND DYSOSTOSES *(contd)*
(Listed in Alphabetical Order)

Disorder	Sex Pre-dominance	Dwarfism	Clinical Features	Abnormalities of Other Tissue Systems	Radiological Features	Remarks
Spondyloepiphyseal Dysplasia—tarda form, 172	Males only	No dwarfism of extremities. Short spine	Milder manifestations and later clinical onset than other two forms. Usually apparent by age 10 years. Children initially normal. Growth of trunk lags behind extremities. Spine short, chest deep and extremities normal in length. Abnormalities of hips often with early degenerative joint disease		Platyspondyly greatest in thoracic area. Pathognomonic configuration of vertebral bodies with hyperostotic new bone formation of posterior two-thirds of articular surfaces. Depression anterior third of vertebral bodies. Narrowing and calcification of disc spaces and spondylotic bridging characterise later stages of disorder. Femoral heads flattened with premature degenerative joint disease. Dysplastic changes in other major joints	Sex-linked recessively-transmitted disorder
Spondylometaphyseal Dysplasia—Kozlowski type, 179		Short-limbed	Recognition mainly in pre-school age with children normal during infancy. Short trunk, short hands and short feet with normal limbs. Varus deformities knees and hips, kyphosis, waddling gait and stiffness of joints. Vision, hearing and intelligence normal		Generalised platyspondyly with increased AP and lateral diameters of vertebral bodies and anterior concavities. Kyphosis common. Odontoid hypoplasia occasionally. Metaphyses of long bones and short, tubular bones broad irregular and sclerotic epiphyseal plates slightly widened. Carpal and tarsal bones develop late. Epiphyseal centres normal. Iliac bones shortened with increased greater sciatic notch and horizontal acetabula. Proximal femoral metaphyses grossly irregular	Inheritance by autosomal dominant mode. Spondylometaphyseal dysplasias (SMD) comprise group of disorders which have in common abnormal metaphyseal and vertebral ossification. Sporadic reports of one or two cases of other types in addition to types Kozlowski and Murdoch
Spondylometaphyseal Dysplasia—Murdoch type, 179		Short-limbed	Short trunk and short limbs at birth, prominent sternum with flaring or lower ribs, bowing of upper extremities, laxity of ligaments around multiple joints and simple pes planus. Growth remains retarded		May resemble Kozlowski type	Differential diagnosis of entities rests generally with poorly defined group of spondyloepiphyseal dysplasia (SED) and metaphyseal chondrodysplasias. In latter, spine changes absent or less prominent. In SED group recognisable epiphyseal as well as metaphyseal abnormalities
Thanatophoric dwarfism (lethal), 141		Neonatal short-limbed dwarfs	Foetus often stillborn. Death from respiratory embarrassment usually occurs within a few hours or days. Infants hypotonic with trunk of normal length, with markedly shortened extremities and relatively large head with prominent forehead. Thorax constricted, abdomen protuberant, arms extended and thighs abducted and externally rotated		Changes in spine characteristic—extreme generalised platyspondyly with large intervertebral spaces, narrow interpedicular distances, particularly in mid-lumbar spine. Small thorax with short horizontal ribs with cupped anterior ends. Small scapulae with normal clavicles. Iliac bones show vertical shortening but are wide horizontally. Acetabula flat and sacrosciatic notches small. Pubic bones short and broad. Clover-leaf anomaly of skull. Long bones usually bowed, short and broad with flaring of metaphyses. Thorn-like projections in metaphyseal areas	Radiological features sufficiently distinctive to permit prenatal diagnosis

B. CONSTITUTIONAL DISEASES OF BONE WITH KNOWN PATHOGENESIS—MUCOPOLYSACCHARIDOSES

Disorder	Clinical Features	Metabolic Error	Genetics	Radiological Features	Remarks
Mucopolysaccharidoses, 120 (seven types which follow)	All types show varying degrees dwarfism with short limbs and spinal abnormalities. Other systems often affected	MPS groups are lysosomal disorders with absence of certain enzymes involved in degradation of specific mucopolysaccharides	Vary	Specific diagnosis may be suggested in many cases. In others, however, specificity very difficult, and additional clinical, biochemical data necessary. Prenatal diagnosis sometimes possible by analysis of fibroblasts cultured from foetal cells obtained from amniotic fluid	Clinical and radiological features must always be correlated with genetic and biochemical studies. Genetic counselling important to forecast prognosis and potential complications

TABLE IB. *Generalised Congenital Disorders (contd.)*

B. CONSTITUTIONAL DISEASES OF BONE WITH KNOWN PATHOGENESIS—MUCOPOLYSACCHARIDOSES *(contd.)*

Disorder	Clinical Features	Metabolic Error	Genetics	Radiological Features	Remarks
MPS I-H—Hurler syndrome, 121	Early clouding cornea, grave manifestations. Mental deterioration after 1-3 years. Contractures, hernia, cardiomegaly, repeated pneumonias. Death by age 10-15 years	Excessive urinary MPS—dermatan sulphate and heparan sulphate Substance deficient—X-L iduronidase (formerly called Hurler corrective factor)	Homozygous for MPS I-H gene	*Skull*—normal at birth. Earliest changes after six months—frontal 'bossing', calvarial thickening, deepening of optic chiasm. Premature fusion sagittal and lambdoidal sutures. Evidence of communicating hydrocephalus. Elongated sella with undermining anterior clinoid processes. Facial bones relatively small. Mandibular angle widened with underdevelopment of condyles. Poorly positioned and malformed teeth. Progressive narrowing nasopharyngeal airway. *Spine.* Thoracolumbar kyphosis, hypoplasia of anterosuperior aspect of first two lumbar vertebrae. Pedicles long and slender. Spatulate rib configuration. *Pelvis.* Widely flared iliac wings and constriction of iliac bones. Coxa valga. *Hands.* Metacarpals and phalanges short and wide with cortical thinning. Bases of metacarpals tapered. Carpal bones small and irregular with delayed maturation. Contracted claw hand occasionally	
MPS I-S (Scheie syndrome), 121	Coarse facies, stiff joints, cloudy cornea, aortic regurgitation, normal intelligence, normal life span. Carpal tunnel syndrome common	Excessive urinary MPS—dermatan sulphate, heparan sulphate Substance deficient—X-L iduronidase	Homozygous for MPS I-S gene	Skeleton may be normal at birth. Slight flattening of vertebral bodies, widening anterior ends of ribs, shafts of long bones and medial portions of clavicles. Carpal bones hypoplastic. Metacarpals shortened with cystic lesions	
MPS I-H/S (Hurler-Scheie compound), 121	Phenotype intermediate between MPS I-H and MPS I-S	Excessive urinary MPS—dermatan sulphate Substance deficient—X-L iduronidase	Genetic compound of MPS I-H and I-S genes	Reminiscent of MPS II group	
MPS II-A—Hunter syndrome, severe, 121	Milder course than in MPS I-H but death usually before age of 15 years. Coarsening of facial features, dwarfism, mental deterioration, flexion deformities and stiff joints. Hepatosplenomegaly, cardiomegaly and early death. Deafness in 50%. Corneal clouding not clinically manifest, although slit lamp examination may disclose opacities	Excessive urinary MPS—dermatan sulphate, heparan sulphate Substance deficient—Hunter corrective factor	Homozygous for X-linked gene	Generally less severe than in individuals in MPS I group. Skull tends to be similar in appearance. Vertebral bodies tend to show less concavity anteriorly and posteriorly and may be slightly diminished in height. Anterior beaking mild; gibbus rare. Flaring of iliac wings of pelvis less prominent; iliac bodies minimally hypoplastic. Coxa valga mild or absent. Ribs may be widened anteriorly. Modelling abnormalities of ribs, long bones and tubular bones of hands generally less severe than in MPS I group	
MPS II-B—Hunter syndrome, mild, 121	Generally less involvement than MPS II-A and often survival to the fourth decade of life or later. Intelligence fair	Excessive urinary MPS—dermatan sulphate, heparan sulphate Substance deficient—Hunter corrective factor	Homozygous for X-linked allele	Similar to MPS II-A (severe form), but less marked	
MPS III-A—Sanfilippo syndrome A, 121	Affected children appear normal first 4 to 5 years of age and then develop progressive, profound, mental deterioration. Physical findings mild, including stiffness of joints, minimal coarsening of features, clawed hands and hepatosplenomegaly. Corneal clouding does not occur	Excessive urinary MPS—heparan sulphate Substance deficient—heparan sulphate sulphatase	Homozygous for Sanfilippo A gene	Skeletal abnormalities mild and variable. Appearance of skull characteristic: hyperostosis parietal and occipital bones and nonpneumatised mastoids. Vertebral bodies slightly increased in AP diameters with minimal anterior beaking	
MPS III-B—Sanfilippo syndrome B, 121	Indistinguishable from MPS III-A	Excessive urinary MPS—heparan sulphate Substance deficient—N-acetyl-z-D-glucosaminidase	Homozygous for Sanfilippo B (at different locus)	Indistinguishable from MPS III-A	

TABLE IB. *Generalised Congenital Disorders (contd.)*

B. CONSTITUTIONAL DISEASES OF BONE WITH KNOWN PATHOGENESIS MUCOPOLYSACCHARIDOSES (*contd.*)

Disorder	Clinical Features	Metabolic Error	Genetics	Radiological Features	Remarks
MPS IV—Morquio's syndrome (probably more than one allelic form), 121	Children normal at birth with distinctive skeletal changes demonstrable in first 18 months. Weakness, hypotonia, kyphosis, frequent respiratory infections, severe dwarfism, lumbar lordosis, severe genu valgum, deformed hands with ulnar deviation. Short nose, wide mouth, dysplastic teeth. Normal intelligence. Corneal opacities. Progressive deafness, atlanto-axial dislocation with paraplegia and respiratory paralysis. Patients may live to adulthood	Excessive urinary MPS—keratan sulphate Substance deficient—unknown	Homozygous for Morquio gene. Transmitted as autosomal recessive trait	Specific diagnostic changes in spine, pelvis, wrists, hands and teeth. Anterior beaking lower thoracic and upper lumbar vertebrae. Hypoplastic odontoid process. Widened intervertebral disc spaces. Flattened vertebral bodies, persistent widening of intervertebral discs. Broadening of anterior ends of ribs with severe pectus carinatum and failure of fusion of sternal segments. Iliac bones severely constricted. Subluxation of hips and coxa valga. Short bones of forearm with widening of proximal ends. Pointing of bases of metacarpals. Delay in appearance and irregularity of carpal centres. Short metacarpals, ulnar deviation of hand. Irregularity of tarsal bones	
MPS V— vacant					
MPS VI-A— Maroteaux-Lamy syndrome, classic form, 121	Resembles MPS I in severity although intelligence normal except in late stages. Survival longer than in MPS I although shorter than in MPS I-S. Prominence of forehead and sternal protrusion at birth. Ultimate dwarfism, short limbs, joint stiffness, lumbar kyphosis, coarsening of facial features, hepatosplenomegaly, corneal clouding and hearing defects common	Excessive urinary MPS—dermatan sulphate Substance deficient —Maroteaux-Lamy corrective factor	Homozygous for M-L gene	May resemble those of MPS I. Dochcephalic skull with enlarged sella and deepened optic chiasm. Premature fusion of sutures Spinal abnormalities generally minimal. Vertebral bodies may show concavities anterior and posterior surfaces and convex superior and inferior surfaces. Anterior beaking of L1 and L2. Hypoplastic odontoid Innominate bone involvement severe—mildly flared iliac wings and constriction of iliac bodies with oblique acetabular roofs. Underdevelopment of ischii and pubic bones. Deficient ossification femoral heads Widening of anterior ends of ribs with small and triangular scapulae and hypoplasia glenoid fossae—subluxation Diaphyseal widening and metaphyseal constriction of long bones. Bowing of radius and ulna. Widening epiphyseal plates and metaphyseal defects. Tubular bones of hands short with modelling abnormalities	
MPS VI-B— Maroteaux-Lamy syndrome, mild form, 121	Milder skeletal and corneal change, normal intellect	Excessive urinary MPS—dermatan sulphate Substance deficient —Maroteaux-Lamy corrective factor	Homozygous for allele at M-L locus	Less severe manifestations than MPS VI-A group	
MPS VII (beta glucuronidase deficiency)—more than one allelic form, 121	Growth retardation, hepatosplenomegaly, impaired mental development, frequent pulmonary infections	Excessive urinary MPS—dermatan sulphate, chondroitin sulphate A and chondroitin sulphate C Substance deficient —beta glucuronidase	Homozygous for mutant gene at beta-glucuronidase locus	Progressive dysostosis multiplex with enlarged skull, prematurely closed sutures and flattened tuberculum sellae. Widened ribs, short rounded scapulae, short wide clavicles, hypoplasia of odontoid process and anterior beaking of lower thoracic and upper lumbar vertebral bodies with kyphosis. Changes in innominate and long bones as in other MPS disorders. Proximal pointing of metacarpals	

C. CONSTITUTIONAL DISEASES OF BONE WITH KNOWN PATHOGENESIS—MUCOLIPIDOSES AND LIPIDOSES

Disorder	Enzyme defect	Excess MPS in Urine	Clinical Features	Radiological Features
GM 1 gangliosidosis—type I, 136	Beta galactosidases A, B, C	None	Severe progressive mental deterioration, psychomotor retardation and death within second year of life. Hepatomegaly, coarse facies, stiff joints, blindness, deafness and disabling rigidity characteristic	Grossly similar to those of MPS I, but earlier and more severe. Periosteal cloaking prominent in early infancy
GM 1 gangliosidosis—type II, 136	Beta galactosidases A, B	None	In early infancy children are normal. Progressive mental and psychomotor retardation from age 6 to 12 months with death generally by age of 10 years	Skeletal changes resemble many of the MPS disorders but tend to be mild
Fucosidosis, 136	Alpha L-fucosidase	None	Cerebral and psychomotor deterioration with myocardial disease beginning at the age of 1 year with death occurring at 4 to 6 years	Minimal skeletal changes resembling very mild forms of MPS disorders A second milder form exists with survival into adulthood

TABLE IB. *Generalised Congenital Disorders (contd.)*

C. CONSTITUTIONAL DISEASES OF BONE WITH KNOWN PATHOGENESIS—MUCOLIPIDOSES AND LIPIDOSES *(contd.)*

Disorder	Enzyme defect	Excess MPS in Urine	Clinical Features	Radiological Features
Mannosidosis, 136	Alpha mannosidase	None	Hepatomegaly and hypotonia evidenced soon after birth. Delay in psychomotor development with mild MPS I-like features. Death generally due to respiratory infection before age of 5 years	Skeletal features resemble mild cases of MPS I
Juvenile sulphatidosis, Austin type, 136	Arylsulphatase A, B, C	Dermatan sulphate, keratan sulphate, sulphatides	Retardation in psychomotor and mental development from birth onward. At age of 2 years progressive deterioration begins and usually death before puberty. Minimal physical findings reminiscent of MPS I disorder	Resemble MPS I disorder from moderate to severe
Mucolipidoses I, 136	Uncertain	None	Early psychomotor development normal, but slowing late in first year with diminution of physical growth. Mild retardation of mental development	Resemble mild manifestations of MPS disorders
Mucolipidosis II (Leroy's I—Cell Disease), 136	Multiple lysosomal enzymes	None	Hurler-like syndrome. Tightness of skin soon after birth, coarse facies, stiffness of joints, failure to thrive, progressive mental deterioration by age of 2 years	Skeletal abnormalities develop early and resemble MPS syndromes may be present at birth. Periosteal cloaking severe
Mucolipidosis III, 136	Multiple lysosomal enzymes	None	Joint stiffness begins from age 1 to 3 years with slow progression to puberty. Retardation of growth leading to dwarfism. Mild mental retardation. Corneal opacities. Coarse facies	Resemble mainly MPS types I or II. In some cases MPS IV and VI in others. Considerable variation in findings
Farber's disease (lipo-granulomatosis), 136	Ceramidase	Dermatan sulphate ceramides	Large granulomatous tumefactions with lipid-containing MPS showing predilection for areas of stress due to motion, e.g. heart, epiglottis, joints. Clinical onset during first few weeks of life with irritability and nodular erythematous joint swellings. Psychomotor and mental retardation with death by 2 years of age	Joint capsule distension, periarticular masses at multiple sites, principally wrists and elbows. Juxta-articular erosions prominent. Resemble MPS syndromes

D. CONSTITUTIONAL DISEASES OF BONE WITH KNOWN PATHOGENESIS—CHROMOSOMAL DISORDERS
(Listed in Alphabetical Order)

Disorder	Sex Predominance	Dwarfism	Clinical Features	Chromosomal Abnormalities	Radiological Features	Remarks
Cri du chat (cat-cry) syndrome, 193		Generalised	Hypoplastic larynx causes characteristic high-pitched cry simulating kitten. Small infants fail to thrive with round facies, microcephaly, antimongoloid palpebral fissures, hypertelorism and low-set ears. Profound mental retardation	Caused by deletion short arm of portion of chromosome—short arm No. 5 (5p-)	Evidence of microcephaly and hypertelorism, short metacarpals, faulty long bone development. Congenital heart disease frequently apparent on film of chest	Diagnosis made clinically and not by radiological criteria. Early disappearance of characteristic cry responsible for lack of specific recognition in older patients
Gonadal dysgenesis (Turner's syndrome), 196	Females	Generalised	Chromosome analyses shows either complete absence of 2nd X chromosome, XO-XX mosaicism or abnormally 2nd X chromosome Sexual infantilism, webbing of neck, sexually immature girls with otherwise normal appearance. Associated cardiovascular and renal anomalies. Occasional mental retardation	XO abnormal chromosome pattern	Skeletal abnormalities varied and inconstant. Retarded bone maturation with short stature. Symmetrical edema of dorsum of each foot may be present in infants. Bilateral cubitus valgus, short third, fourth and fifth metacarpals, premature fusion of ossification centres of metacarpals, enlargement of medial tibial plateau with depression of medial epiphysis and metaphysis and often small exostosis inferiorly. Pes cavus, 'drumstick' distal phalanges of hands, scoliosis, kyphosis, parietal thinning and generalised osteoporosis. Hypoplasia of cervical spine may also occur	Associated cardiovascular (coarctation of aorta and aortic stenosis) and renal anomalies (most common). These anomalies less frequent in chromatin negative XO patients. Mental retardation uncommon compared with Noonan's syndrome
Idiopathic hemi-hypertrophy (asymmetry)			Mental retardation, hypertrophy appendicular skeleton. Skull abnormalities—dolichocephaly or oxycephaly, antimongoloid slant, hyperpigmentation of trunk, syndactyly	Cell cultures of fibroblasts showed 69 chromosomes in some cells in triploid groupings. Sex chromosomes grouped XXY. Fibroblasts mainly diploid, some triploid	Hemihypertrophy appendicular skeleton and even flat bones (pelvis)	Medullary sponge kidney reported with idiopathic hemihypertrophy

TABLE IB. *Generalised Congenital Disorders (contd.)*

D. CONSTITUTIONAL DISEASES OF BONE WITH KNOWN PATHOGENESIS—CHROMOSOMAL DISORDERS
(Listed in Alphabetical Order)

Disorder	Sex Pre-dominance	Dwarfism	Clinical Features	Chromosomal Abnormalities	Radiological Features	Remarks
Klinefelters syndrome (dysgenesis seminiferous tubules)	Males		Small or absent testicles. Gynaeco-mastia-eunuchoid constitution. Main cause of infertility. Urinary gonadotropins rise to high levels after puberty	XXY chromosome pattern. 47 chromosomes with extra X chromosome	No distinctive radiological findings although short 4th metacarpal and small bridged sella turcica have been described	May be commonest chromosomal aberration
Mongolism (Down's syndrome), 192		Generalised	Variable. Mental retardation profound. Hypotonia in infancy with small brachiocephalic head, small mouth, protruding tongue, epicanthal folds, small flat nose, small abnormal teeth and short, wide hands, with short curved 5th fingers. Complex cardiac anomalies present in 50 to 75% of cases—endocardial cushion defect or ventricular septal defects. Increased incidence duodenal atresia or stenosis and aganglionic megacolon	Somatic chromosome abnormality. Trisomy G group, 21-23	Vertebral bodies tall and thin. Microcrania with delayed closing of sutures, brachycephaly, orbital hypertelorism, persistent metopic suture. Hypoplastic facial bones, deformed teeth, gracile ribs, absence 12th ribs occasionally, atlanto-axial subluxation, double ossification centres of manubrium. Pelvic measurements diagnostic with small iliac index. 'Elephant ear' pelvis. Abnormal findings in extremities confined to fingers and toes—hypoplastic middle phalanges and 5th fingers hands with clinodactyly	Single film of pelvis in infant often diagnostic because of abnormal acetabular index. High maternal age. Leukemia in affected child and mother occurs more often than in normal population
Noonan's syndrome, 196	Occurs in both males and females, with normal karyotypes	Generalised but not always present	Webbing of neck, short stature in some but not invariably, abnormal facies including hypertelorism, small mandible with dental occlusion, gonads vary from absent to normal, retarded maturation and delayed puberty occurs. Mental retardation common in contrast to Turner's syndrome	Normal karyotypes	Small mandible, hypertelorism, pectus carinatum and excavatum common. Other skeletal anomalies exist far less frequently than in Turner's syndrome	Renal anomalies less common than in Turner's syndrome. Most often renal malrotation. Cardiac anomalies frequent but different from Turner's syndrome—valvar pulmonic stenosis, atrial septal defects and eccentric hypertrophy of left ventricle. Striking familial incidence
Orodigito-facial syndrome	Females		Mental retardation. Clefts in tongue, palate and jaws. Abnormalities of dentition. Orbital hypertelorism. Deformities of fingers	Autosomal trisomy of No. 1 chromosome. No. of chromosomes 47. Linked with sex chromosomes —lethal in male. Nuclear chromatin pattern usually female	Hypoplasia mandible and occiput of skull. Evidence of cleft palate and cleft in jaw bones. Phalanges shortened but metacarpals may be elongated	Renal polycystic disease may be associated. Some elements of this syndrome found in other congenital conditions, e.g. Ellis-van Creveld syndrome

TABLE IB. *Generalised Congenital Disorders* (*contd.*)

D. CONSTITUTIONAL DISEASES OF BONE WITH KNOWN PATHOGENESIS—CHROMOSOMAL DISORDERS
(Listed in Alphabetical Order)

Disorder	Sex Pre-dominance	Dwarfism	Clinical Features	Chromosomal Abnormalities	Radiological Features	Remarks
Trisomy D (13-15) syndrome, 193			Infants hypertonic and severely retarded mentally. Most die within 6 months. Microcephaly, cleft palate and lip, hypotelorism, colobomata, cataracts, micro-ophthalmia, malformed ears with hypoplastic external auditory canals common. Polydactyly and hyperconvex nails and heels prominent in appendicular skeleton. Associated anomalies include capillary hemangioma on face and upper trunk. Various cardiac, genitourinary, gastrointestinal and central nervous system anomalies, particularly of the holo-prosencephalic type	Karyotype shows an additional chromosome in D group	Deficient ossification of skull with evidence of arhinencephaly. Cleft or absent midline structures of facial bones, poorly formed orbits and slanting frontal bones. Thin malformed ribs and often diaphragmatic hernia and evidence of congenital heart disease. Most common finding in hand is post-axial polydactyly. Other radiological features reflect various anomalies	Death in infancy usual. High maternal age. Post-axial polydactyly diagnostic radiologically
Trisomy 18 syndrome (E Trisomy), 192	Usually female	Generalised	Hypertonic infants. Mental and psychomotor retardation. Facies typical with micrognathia, close-set ears, high, narrow palate. Flexed, ulnar-deviated fingers and short adducted thumb, with characteristic finding of second finger overlapping third. Short first toe and 'rocker bottom' foot deformities frequent. Congenital heart disease almost invariably present—ventricular septal defect and patent ductus arteriosus. Other anomalies—gastrointestinal and renal—may also occur. Usually die before age of six months	An additional chromosome at 18 or E group location	Thin calvaria, hypoplastic maxilla and mandible, gracile ribs, hypoplastic sternum and clavicles. Iliac bones rotated anteriorly with increased obliquity of acetabulae. Short first metacarpals and phalanges, ulnar deviation of fingers, short first toes, 'rocker bottom' deformity of feet and extreme pes planus. Evidence of congenital heart disease of various types in film of chest. Diaphragmatic eventration common	Short adducted thumb and overlap of second on third finger diagnostic radiologically

REPORT OF THE 'COMMITTEE ON NOMENCLATURE OF INTRINSIC DISEASES OF BONE'

Fauré, C., Kaufmann, H. J., Kozlowski, K., Langer, L. O., Lefèbvre, J., Maroteaux, P., Sauvegrain, J., Silverman, F. N., Spranger, J.

CONSTITUTIONAL (INTRINSIC) DISEASES OF BONES

Constitutional Diseases of Bones with Unknown Pathogenesis

Osteochondrodysplasia
(abnormalities of cartilage and/or bone growth and development)

1. *Defects of growth or tubular bones and/or spine*

    A—*Manifested at birth*
    1. Achondrogenesis
    2. Thanatophoric dwarfism
    3. Achondroplasia
    4. Chondrodysplasia punctata (formerly stippled epiphyses) (several forms)
    5. Metatropic dwarfism
    6. Diastrophic dwarfism
    7. Chondro-ectodermal dysplasia (Ellis-Van Creveld)
    8. Asphyxiating thoracic dysplasia (Jeune)
    9. Spondylo-epiphyseal dysplasia congenita
    10. Mesomelic dwarfism: type Nievergelt; type Langer
    11. Cleido-cranial dysplasia (formerly cleido-cranial dysostosis)

    B—*Manifested in later life*

    1. Hypochondroplasia
    2. Dyschondrosteosis
    3. Metaphyseal chondro-dysplasia type Jansen
    4. Metaphyseal chondro-dysplasia type Schmid
    5. Metaphyseal chondro-dysplasia type McKusick (formerly cartilage-hair-hypoplasia)
    6. Metaphyseal chondro-dysplasia with mal-absorption and neutropenia
    7. Metaphyseal chondro-dysplasia with thymo-lymphopenia
    8. Spondylo-metaphyseal dysplasia (Kozlowski)
    9. Multiple epiphyseal dysplasia (several forms)
    10. Hereditary arthro-ophthalmopathy
    11. Pseudo-achondroplasic dysplasia (formerly spondylo-epiphyseal pseudo-achondroplasic dysplasia)
    12. Spondylo-epiphyseal dysplasia tarda
    13. Acrodysplasia
        Rhino-tricho-phalangeal syndrome (Giedion)
        Epiphyseal (Thiemann)
        Epiphyso-metaphyseal (Brailsford)

2. *Disorganised development of cartilage and fibrous components of the skeleton*
    1. Dysplasia epiphysealis hemimelica
    2. Multiple cartilagenous exostoses
    3. Enchondromatosis (Ollier's disease)
    4. Enchondromatosis with hemangioma (Maffucci's syndrome)
    5. Fibrous dysplasia (Jaffe-Lichtenstein)
    6. Fibrous dysplasia with skin pigmentation and precocious puberty (McCune-Albright)
    7. Cherubism
    8. Multiple fibromatosis

3. *Abnormalities of density, of cortical diaphyseal structure and/or of metaphyseal modelling*
    1. Osteogenesis imperfecta congenita (Vrolik, Porak-Durante)
    2. Osteogenesis imperfecta tarda (Lobstein)
    3. Juvenile idiopathic osteoporosis
    4. Osteopetrosis with precocious manifestations
    5. Osteopetrosis with delayed manifestations
    6. Pycnodysostosis
    7. Osteopoikilosis
    8. Melorheostosis
    9. Diaphyseal dysplasia (Camurati-Engelmann)
    10. Cranio-diaphyseal dysplasia
    11. Endosteal hyperostosis (Van Buchem and other forms)
    12. Tubular stenosis (Kenny-Caffey)
    13. Osteodysplastia
    14. Pachydermoperiostosis
    15. Osteo-ectasia with hyperphosphatasia
    16. Metaphyseal dysplasia (Pyle's disease)
    17. Cranio-metaphyseal dysplasia (several forms)
    18. Fronto-metaphyseal dysplasia
    19. Oculo-dental-osseous dysplasia (formerly oculo-dento-digital syndrome)

Dysostosis
(Malformation of individual bones, single or in combination)

1. *Dystostosis with cranial and facial involvement*
    1. Craniosynostosis, several forms
    2. Cranio-facial dysostosis (Crouzon)
    3. Acrocephalo-syndactylia (Apert)
    4. Acrocephalo-polysyndactylia (Carpenter)
    5. Mandibulo-facial dysostosis (Treacher-Collins, Franceschetti and others)

6. Mandibular hypoplasia (includes Pierre Robin syndrome)
7. Oculo-mandibulo-facial syndrome (Haller-man-Streiff-François)
8. Nevoid basal cell carcinoma syndrome

2. *Dysostosis with predominant axial involvement*
    1. Vertebral segmentation defects (including Klippel-Feil)
    2. Cervico-oculo-acoustic syndrome (Wilder-vank)
    3. Sprengel's deformity
    4. Spondylo-costal dysostosis (several forms)
    5. Oculo-vertebral syndrome (Weyers)
    6. Osteo-onychodysostosis (formerly nail-patella-syndrome)

3. *Dystostosis with predominant involvement of extremities*
    1. Amelia
    2. Hemimelia (several types)
    3. Acheiria
    4. Apodia
    5. Adactylia and oligadactylia
    6. Phocomelia
    7. Aglossia-adactylia syndrome
    8. Congenital bowing of long bones (several types)
    9. Familial radio-ulnar synostosis
    10. Brachydactylia (several types)
    11. Symphalangism
    12. Polydactylia (several types)
    13. Syndactylia (several types)
    14. Poly-syndactylia (several types)
    15. Camptodactylia
    16. Clinodactylia
    17. Laurence-Moon syndrome
    18. Popliteal pterygium syndrome
    19. Pectoral aplasia—dysdactylia syndrome (Poland)
    20. Rubinstein-Taybi syndrome
    21. Pancytopenia—dysmelia syndrome (Fanconi)
    22. Thrombocytopenia—radial aplasia syndrome
    23. Oro-digito-facial syndrome (Papillon-Leage)
    24. Cardiomelique syndrome (Holt, Oram and others)

Idiopathic Osteolysis

Acro-osteolysis:
    phalangeal type
    tarso-carpal form with or without nephropathy
Multicentric osteolysis

Primary Disturbances of Growth
    1. Primordial dwarfism (without associated malformation)
    2. Cornelia de Lange's syndrome
    3. Bird-headed dwarfism (Virchow, Seckel)
    4. Leprechaunism
    5. Russell-Silver syndrome
    6. Progeria
    7. Cockayne's syndrome
    8. Bloom's syndrome
    9. Geroderma osteodysplastica
    10. Spherophakia—Brachymorphia syndrome (Weill-Marchesani)
    11. Marfan's syndrome

Constitutional Diseases of Bones with Known Pathogenesis

Chromosomal Aberrations

PRIMARY METABOLIC ABNORMALITIES

1. *Calcium-phosphorus metabolism*
    1. Hypophosphatemic familial rickets
    2. Pseudo-deficiency rickets (type Royer, Prader)
    3. Late rickets (type McCance)
    4. Idiopathic hypercalciuria
    5. Hypophosphatasia (several forms)
    6. Idiopathic hypercalcemia
    7. Pseudo-hypoparathyroidism (Normo- and hypercalcemic forms)

2. *Mucopolysaccharidosis*
    1. Mucopolysaccharidosis I (Hurler)
    2. Mucopolysaccharidosis II (Hunter)
    3. Mucopolysaccharidosis III (Sanfilippo)
    4. Mucopolysaccharidosis IV (Morquio)
    5. Mucopolysaccharidosis V (Ullrich-Scheie)
    6. Mucopolysaccharidosis VI (Maroteaux-Lamy)

3. *Mucolipidosis and lipidosis*
    1. Mucolipidosis I (Spranger-Wiedemann)
    2. Mucolipidosis II (Leroy)
    3. Mucolipidosis III (Pseudo-polydystrophy)
    4. Fucosidosis
    5. Mannosidosis
    6. Generalised GM, gangliosidosis (several forms)
    7. Sulfatidosis with mucopolysacchariduria (Austin, Thieffry)
    8. Cerebrosidosis including Gaucher's disease

4. *Other metabolic extra-osseous disorders*

BONY ABNORMALITIES SECONDARY TO DISTURBANCES OF EXTRA-SKELETAL SYSTEMS
    1. Endocrine
    2. Hematologic
    3. Neurologic
    4. Renal
    5. Gastro-intestinal
    6. Cardio-pulmonary

TABLE IC. *Scoliosis*

Type	Age and Sex	Cause	Characteristic Features	Remarks
Postural, 990	Children and adults	Faulty posture, shortening of limb, sciatic list, hysteria	Correctable list of spine. Usually transient	May become fixed (structural) if not corrected
Idiopathic—infantile, 991	Infancy. Slightly more common in boys	Unknown	Curves usually convex to left. Have progressive and spontaneously resolving types. Require evaluation R-V angle difference to determine prognosis (see text)	Virtually unknown North American continent. Common in Great Britain
Idiopathic—juvenile and adolescent, 991	Childhood and adolescence. Multi-factorial mode of inheritance (?)	Unknown. ? Congenital	Four types of curves: thoracic, lumbar, thoraco-lumbar and combined thoracic and lumbar	May lead to impairment pulmonary function. May be associated with congenital heart disorders
Congenital, 998	Usually early childhood	Congenital	Two broad groups: errors of development and errors of segmentation *Errors of development*: spina bifida, butterfly vertebrae, hemivertebrae *Errors of segmentation*: Unilateral failure of segmentation May be associated with rib anomalies. Degree and type of scoliosis varies	Spinal dysraphism is special form—midline errors of development of back, e.g. tethered cord, diastematomyelia, intra-spinal lipoma This group associated frequently with congenital anomalies genito-urinary, central nervous and cardio-vascular systems and other skeletal anomalies
Scoliosis associated with cerebral palsy, 1001	Early childhood	Muscle paresis	Curves initially mild and of paralytic long C pattern	Curves may progress rapidly
Scoliosis associated with spinal and peripheral neuromuscular disorder, 1000	Generally in childhood but may occur in adults. Depends on cause	Large number of disorders—genetic and acquired (see text)	Type, degree and extent of curves vary with cause. Usually develops some years after onset of disorder. Two major types of scoliosis: long C curve—thoracic and lumbar although entire spine may be affected; thoracic and lumbar combined curves	Rotation present to moderate or marked degree. Usually progressive
Painful scoliosis, 1006	Varies with cause—usually children and young adults	Multiple, e.g. osteoid osteoma, osteoblastoma, aneurysmal bone cyst, osteomyelitis, eosinophil granuloma. Due to muscle spasm	Lesion present on *concave* side of scoliotic curve with curve *convex* to opposite side	Presence of scoliosis accompanied by localised pain. Often necessitates tomography to establish identity of causative lesion
Scoliosis associated with connective tissue disorders, 1008	Generally infants and young children	Multiple. Include chromosomal disorders and various skeletal dysplasias (see text)	May have kyphosis in addition to scoliosis. Type of curve variable	An extensive list of heritable disorders producing scoliosis now appreciated

TABLE IIA. *Acute Trauma*

Site	Special Features of Interest
1. Skull, 202	Any bone of skull may be affected. Basal skull fractures particularly important. Horizontal lateral film essential Usually, diagnosis of skull fracture of limited value to clinician; does not necessarily reveal condition of patient. Severe intracranial damage may occur in absence of fracture and conversely normal examination does not exempt patient from neurological complications. Pneumocephalus a possible complication
2. Facial bones, 203	'Blow-out' fracture of orbit occurs due to fracture of Orbital wall. Inferior rectus muscle may herniate through orbital floor, producing soft tissue mass radiologically Fractures of facial bones generally result from direct frontal injuries. Include fractures of nose and zygomatic arch LeFort classification: *LeFort I* —low transverse fractures; *LeFort II* —pyramidal fractures; *LeFort III*—high transverse fracture Fractures of mandible result from indirect violence generally; often both sides fracture. Fractures of angle and body of mandible common. Fractures of neck and mandibular condyle difficult to demonstrate. May be intracapsular or extracapsular. Intracapsular fracture may be associated with dislocation of condyle
3. Cervical spine, 204	Hyperflexion and hyperextension forces generally responsbile for injury to cervical vertebrae. Hyperflexion results in compression or vertical fracture of vertebral body. More severe hyperflexion—separation of spinous process at one or more levels with dislocation of articular facets Fractures and dislocations in atlanto-axial region and posterior arch of atlas important. *Jefferson* fracture is bursting fracture of atlas. Direct injury may result in fracture of spinous process and posterior part of vertebral arch. Brachial plexus avulsions may produce traumatic meningocoeles, **259** Forced hyperextension may result in rupture of anterior spinal ligament, separation of adjoining vertebral bodies and compression of posterior elements of vertebra Films may be essentially normal yet may have severe compression damage to cord
4. Pectoral girdle and shoulder, 209	Clavicular fracture common—due to fall on outstretched hand. Acromioclavicular joint frequent site of dislocation. Anterior dislocation of humeral head much more common than posterior dislocation, which is often associated with injuries related to muscle spasm. Generally result of uncoordinated muscle contractions—epilepsy, tetanus, accidental electric shock. Dislocation of humeral head often results in compression fracture—*Hill-Sachs* or *Bankhart* detect. Calcification or ossification of coracoclavicular ligament often late sequel to acromioclavicular separation
5. Neck of humerus, 212	Comminuted fracture due to direct injury. Generally results in fracture of greater tuberosity and fissure fracture across surgical neck. In adduction fractures of surgical neck shaft adducted in relation to humeral head. Abduction fracture of surgical neck often results in associated fracture-separation of greater tuberosity. Small number of fractures of proximal end of humerus often comminuted with separation and displacement of either tuberosity
6. Elbow, 213	Supracondylar fracture of humerus most common elbow fracture in children. 'Fat-pad' sign important—particularly posterior 'fat pad'. May also indicate fracture of radial head. If capsule is torn fat pad sign often absent. Adult equivalent of childhood supracondylar fracture may produce extension into elbow joint. Fractures of both humeral condyles occur at any age. Fracture-separation of medial epicondyle important injury to recognise. Fragment may be separated into joint. Important to assess relationship of radial head to capitulum in children. Fracture through trochlear notch of olecranon involves joint surface—usually result of direct blow Fractures of upper end of radius may involve head or neck. Radial neck fracture frequent in immature skeleton—often an epiphyseal fracture—separation. Posterior dislocation of ulna result of considerable force—generally associated with avulsion fracture coronoid process of ulna Dislocation of radial head uncommon as isolated injury; may be associated with fracture of ulnar shaft (*Monteggia injury*)
7. Forearm and wrist, 216, 217	Fracture single bone of forearm rare as isolated injury. Fracture upper half of ulnar shaft associated with radial head dislocation (*Monteggia injury*). Fracture of distal half radial shaft often combined with dislocation distal radio-ulnar joint (*Galeazzi injury*) Fractures around wrist include *Colles* fracture—distal end of radius with backward and lateral displacement of distal fragment radius. In fracture of distal end of radius anterior displacement of distal fragment characteristic of *Smith* fracture. In children, fracture-separation of distal radial epiphysis represents counterpart of Colles and Smith fractures
8. Carpus, 218, 219	Commonest injury—fracture of scaphoid in adolescent or young adult. Three types—waist, tubercle, proximal pole. Fractures of waist and proximal pole liable to development of post-traumatic necrosis Triquetrum is next most commonly fractured carpal bone, generally identified as flake of bone detached from posterior-medial surface in lateral view Perilunar dislocation of carpus consists of several types. Actual dislocation of lunate much less commonly encountered (see text)
9. Thoracic and lumbar spine and thorax, 222, 257	Fractures of thoracic spine usually result from hyperflexion injury with resultant compression and anterior wedging of vertebral bodies. Comminuted fractures of vertebral arches may occur. Fracture-dislocation of lumbar spine not uncommon and generally unstable. Generally results from hyperflexion injuries, often resulting in neurological deficits. Seat-belt syndrome refers to combination of injuries to spinal column, pelvic girdle and thorax, together with flexion injuries to lumbar spine. Fractures of lumbar transverse processes may be unassociated with other skeletal injuries sustained during falls. Represent basically avulsion injuries due to avulsion of ligaments and intertransverse muscles. Isolated or associated fractures of ribs may cause pneumothorax, pulmonary contusion syndrome and other pulmonary complications

TABLE IIA. *Acute Trauma* (*contd.*)

Site	Special Features of Interest
10. Pelvis and acetabulum, 229	Divided into three groups: (1) fracture-dislocations of pelvic ring due to crushing injury; (2) avulsion fractures of muscle attachments; and (3) fractures of sacrum and coccyx Pelvic ring injuries may be divided into fractures of pubic rami, fractures through body of ilium and diastasis of pubic symphysis or sacro-iliac joint. Important to exclude injury at another point in bony wing, when fracture or dislocation is identified, e.g. diastasis at pubic symphysis with fractures of the pubic rami often combined with dislocations of sacro-iliac joint and fracture through body of ilium. Isolated fractures of sacrum and coccyx generally result from falls
11. Hip, 226	Posterior dislocation of hip much more common than anterior dislocation; may result occasionally in post-traumatic necrosis. Central dislocation of femoral head basically a fracture of central region of acetabulum
12. Proximal portion of femur, 232	Fractures around femoral neck very common. Particularly in older people, usually associated with osteoporosis or osteomalacia. Fractures of femoral neck divided into intracapsular and extracapsular varieties. Ischaemic necrosis of femoral head frequent complication of intracapsular fractures (15-20%), regardless of type or competence of treatment
13. Trochanters, 232	Either trochanter may be involved in avulsion injury. Fracture of femoral neck in children results in high incidence ischaemic necrosis femoral head. Fractures of proximal shaft of femur below trochanters usually result in separation of bone ends with associated muscle injury
14. Knee, 240	Supracondylar fractures of femur relatively uncommon. Osteochondral fractures of femoral condyles common in adolescence—due to severe, combined, rotatory compression force. *Salter* classification applied to epiphyseal plate injuries: Salter type I—separation of whole epiphysis with peripheral fragment of metaphyses attached to epiphyses; Salter type II—fracture-separation of epiphysis with peripheral fragment of metaphysis attached to epiphysis; Salter type III—only part of epiphysis is separated, with fracture line extending from articular surface to growth plate and cortex; Salter type IV—fracture line extends through the joint surface across growth plate, shearing off portion of metaphysis; Salter type V—results from severe compression force with crushing effect on epiphyseal plate—relatively uncommon with poor prognosis (premature fusion) Bumper or fender fracture represents valgus strain, rupturing medial ligament and involving femoral condyle with impingement on tibial plateau, causing depressed fracture. Also associated fracture of neck of fibula. Ruptured cruciate ligaments and vertical fracture of tibial condyle can also occur Complete dislocation of knee joint indicates rupture of collateral and cruciate ligaments in addition to joint capsule
15. Patella, 235	Patella generally fractured by direct violence, usually producing transverse, comminuted or, rarely, vertical fracture line. Dislocation of patella may be congenital or traumatic. Osteochondral fractures may result because of excursion of patella
16. Ankle, 242	*Pott's* fractures—fracture-dislocation divided into three degrees: First degree—fracture involving one malleolus only—either lateral or medial; Second degree—unstable fracture with one or two malleoli involved and complete rupture of collateral ligament; Third degree—trimalleolar fracture. Adduction injuries least common Abduction fracture-dislocations result from stress on inferior tibial-fibular ligament, provided distal portion of fibula remains intact. Diastasis occurs in tibial-fibular joint if ligament ruptures In all ankle injuries important to assess ankle mortice—relationship of talus to tibia
17. Tarsus, 246	In fractures of calcaneus evaluation of Böhler's angle in lateral film important. Separation of bony fragments from calcaneal tuberosity and anterior margin of sustentaculum tali may occur
18. Talus, 246	Can result from dorsiflexion force applied to foot which may fracture neck of talus. Associated dislocation of tibiotalar or tibiocalcaneal joint or both may occur. Dislocation of talonavicular joint also possible
19. Navicular, 246	Fractures generally avulsive in type and often incidental to injuries such as ankle sprain or fracture-dislocation. Fragments avulsed from superior surface of navicular in forced plantar flexion injury. Avulsion fractures of tuberosities of navicular may occur. Transverse fracture of navicular uncommon, resulting from compression of bone between talus and cuneiforms in dorsiflexion. May be accompanied by talonavicular subluxation *Lisfranc* fracture-dislocations—represent tarsometatarsal injuries. Base of second metatarsal often fractured *Robert Jones* fracture (fracture base of 5th metatarsal) is common injury generally associated with forced inversion of foot, resulting from avulsion of tubercle of metatarsal by attached tendon of peroneus brevis muscle

TABLE IIB. *Other Traumatic Lesions of the Skeleton*

Sub-group	Sites of Predilection	Special Features of Interest	Complications	Remarks
1. Lesions due to chronic stress *a.* **Stress or fatigue fractures** *b.* **Stress reactions, 262**	Second metatarsal neck, tibia, calcaneus, femoral neck, pars interarticularis of neural arch (may cause spondylolisthesis) Iliac component of sacroiliac joints (osteitis condensans ilii). Anterior cortex of tibia	Lesions may only become apparent by callus formation some days after onset of pain. Frequently associated with specific activity In osteitis condensans ilii dense subchondral sclerosis. Occurs bilaterally in women and attributed to parturition stress. Regresses and not observed in elderly Anterior cortex of tibia thickens with chronic stress. (Ballet dancers and long-distance runners)	Non-union occasionally, especially in mid-shaft of tibia. Chronic stress may thicken anterior tibial cortex Osteitis condensans ilii associated with chronic low back pain Unilateral stress reactions may be seen with chronic disorders of the opposite hip	Callus formation may suggest infection or malignant tumour. Serial studies show organisation and regression Cortical thickening of second metatarsal shaft probably result of unrecognised stress fracture
2. Avulsion injuries, 274	Tendon insertions, ligamentous attachments and muscle origin and insertion sites, e.g. tibial tuberosity (Osgood-Schlatter lesion), anterior inferior spine of ilium (origin of rectus femoris muscle), ischial apophysis (origin of adductor muscles of thigh), lesser trochanter of femur (insertion of psoas muscle), anterior superior iliac spine (origin of sartorius muscle), and distal femoral metaphysis (adductor muscles)—'parosteal desmoid'	*Acute injuries* in adults, e.g. dorsal aspect of navicular in high jumpers *Chronic stress* causes irregularities and new bone formation	Avulsed fragments may never unite and grow to cause large bony excrescences in soft tissues (post-traumatic mineralisation or 'myositis ossificans')	Chronic avulsion injuries formerly described as 'osteochondritis'
3. Joint injuries, 306	Shoulder (especially with recurrent dislocation), knee, ankle, elbow	*Compression injuries* (osteochondral fractures) of convex articular surfaces—humeral head, femoral condyles, capitulum, medial aspect of talus, rarely head of femur after dislocation *Fat-fluid level* in joint always indicates associated bone injury	Inferior subluxation of humeral head common with humeral shaft fractures owing to muscle wasting	Elbow joint effusions displace anterior and posterior fat-pads if capsule intact. Stress changes may affect symphysis pubis
4. Injuries due to muscle spasm, 300	Spine, shoulder (posterior dislocation), neck of femur, patella	Caused by *simple reflex spasm* (patella, olecranon process) and *generalised spasm*—epilepsy, tetanus, electric shock and electroconvulsive therapy, strychnine poisoning and tetany particularly after parathyroidectomy in treatment of hyperparathyroidism	Compression fractures of spine in children may show remarkable regeneration and restoration of shape during remaining years of growth	Paravertebral haematoma around a fracture of thoracic spine may resemble abscess radiologically
5. Soft tissue injuries, 874	Quadriceps and adductor muscles of thigh. Tendons and ligaments around shoulder, knee and ankle. Bursae over bony prominences	Amorphous calcification whose shape may permit identification of anatomical structure affected. Especially common in supraspinatus tendon sheath	Rupture of tendon sheath or bursa may cause diffuse spread of calcified material (and incidentally relieve pain)	Traumatic subperiosteal ossification ('myositis ossificans') in thigh may suggest malignant tumour. Many other causes of calcification but appearance different, e.g. vascular, metabolic, neoplastic, parasitic and paraplegic
6. Post-traumatic necrosis (avascular or aseptic necrosis), 330	(a) *Following frank fracture:* neck of femur, proximal pole of scaphoid, body of talus	Death of bone does not alter radiological appearance unless (1) absorption takes place, (2) revascularisation occurs. The former increases translucency, the latter density, by apposition of new viable bone over dead trabeculae	Fractures of femoral neck in children especially liable to be followed by femoral head necrosis	Compromise of vascular supply on *venous* side may be significant factor in causing necrosis of femoral head after fracture
	(b) *Involving whole bone centre* ('osteochondritis'). Lunate (Kienböck's disease), navicular (Köhler's disease). 2nd metatarsal head (Frieberg's disease). Great toe sesamoid ? femoral head (Perthes' disease), **350**	No specific history of injury. Slow progression of increase of density due to attempted repair and fragmentation. Joint space widening with 'irritable hip' syndrome important as a precursor	Dense bone of repair still weak and subject to collapse and crumbling. Prolonged protection required. Necrotic changes may not become visible for many months after fracture has united, especially in femoral head. Severe cases without prolonged protection usually require arthroplasty or arthrodesis to relieve pain	Differentiate from necrosis of systemic origin; infarction in sickle-cell disease, Gaucher's disease, haemophilia, polycythaemia, and also from caisson disease
	(c) *Involving articular surface* 'osteochondritis dissecans' femoral condyles (König's disease) capitellum, articular surface of talus, 1st metatarsal head	These abnormalities all show defects on a convex articular surface, containing a separate fragment of bone	Fragment of bone or cartilage may separate into joint as loose body, maintain viability through synovial fluid and actually enlarge	These subarticular post-traumatic necroses especially common in athletes, but also appear to be precipitated by minor anatomical abnormalities. Multiple lesions common in late stages of dysplasia epiphysealis multiplex

TABLE IIB. *Other Traumatic Lesions of the Skeleton (contd.)*

Sub-group	Sites of Predilection	Special Features of Interest	Complications	Remarks
7. Perthes' disease, 350	Femoral capital epiphysis	Age of incidence from 2 to 14 years with peak between 4 and 5 years. Males more often than females. Disease bilateral in more than 10%. Initial change—lateral subluxation of femoral head. Subarticular zone of translucency femoral head with subsequent separation of curvilinear fragment. Epiphyseal centre then becomes flattened, fragmented and dense. Changes represent necrosis of bone followed by revascularisation and often slow reformation of femoral head, with residual flattening and widening of femoral neck. Lytic areas in metaphysis represent fibrous tissue or cartilage	Severe secondary degenerative joint disease in adult life	Cause—probably secondary to transient obstruction of venous drainage by mechanical pressure of joint effusion, which may be due to mild trauma or even inflammatory process. Results in compensatory hypervascularity of synovial tissue with hypertrophy
8. Traumatic lesions due to physical agents	*Frostbite* (pernio)-extremities, especially fingers and toes, **344**	Vascular supply destroyed. Bone absorption without reformation. Premature fusion adjacent epiphyses in children	Loss of digits and hypoplasia of remainder if growth incomplete	Other forms of acro-osteolysis include Raynaud's disease and idiopathic type
	Radiation necrosis. Shoulder girdle (after carcinoma of breast); pelvis and hips (after gynecological cancer), **632**	Radiological changes include evidence of bone death (ischemic sequestrum formation, lytic areas, reactive bone sclerosis and secondary calcification), osteoporosis and retardation of bone growth. Premature epiphyseal fusion may occur	Factors which influence clinical radiological patterns of radiation damage include: (1) radiotherapy time—dose relations; (2) area of skeleton being treated; and (3) presence of associated infection, which leads to rapid progression of skeletal changes after radiation. Difficulty may exist in distinguishing radiation osteitis from radiation induced sarcoma	Radium salts were used therapeutically up to 1930 and areas of bone destruction and sclerosis may still be encountered. Necrosis of maxilla and mandible from radioactive paints being licked from the brushes of dial painters now historical
	Dysbaric osteonecrosis (*caisson disease*). Humeral and femoral heads, shafts of long bones, **344**	Too rapid decompression from high atmosphere liberates free nitrogen in blood stream, blocking capillaries and causing infarcts and subarticular necrosis. Areas of irregular density and translucency	Infarcts in shafts unimportant, but subarticular fragments of bone may separate into joint as loose bodies. Secondary degenerative joint disease common	Observed rarely in high-flying aviators without pressurisation
9. Traumatic lesions of neuropathic origin, 378	*Neurosyphilis:* spine, hip, knee, ankle. *Syringomyelia:* shoulder, elbow, wrist, hand. *Congenital absence of pain sense:* lower limbs, hands. *Spina bifida:* ankle and foot. *Diabetic neuropathy:* foot. *Leprosy:* hands and feet. *Paraplegia:* lower limbs	'Charcot' joints, described in 1868, are now considered to be the result of repeated trauma, from which absent or diminished pain sense prevents protection by muscle reflexes. Painless fractures important feature. Joint disorganisations progress at variable rate, numerous fragments of bone being separated and sometimes ground into debris. Subluxations and dislocations eventually develop. In leprosy, joints subject to greatest stress affected most—interphalangeal in hands and metatarsophalangeal in feet. In paraplegia, unfelt fractures may provoke excessive callus formation, possibly resembling tumours	Arthrodesis tends to be unsuccessful, neighbouring joints then being affected. Lesions in foot frequently accompanied by trophic ulcers and secondary infection of bone and soft tissue, again with diminished or absent pain sense. Soft tissue ossification round hips common in paraplegia	Disintegration of joints common in iatrogenic Cushing's syndrome, closely simulating frankly neuropathic variety. Hips and knees mainly affected. Pain sense again diminished and bones osteoporotic, unlike other neuropathic lesions. Similar changes in these joints observed with other forms of pain-relieving therapy in degenerative joint disease, **707, 836**. Rapid progression of skeletal changes in a matter of weeks or months may sometimes occur. In diabetes and syringomyelia superadded infection not uncommon. May then result in juxta-articular osteoporosis, not ordinarily present in neuropathic skeletal disorders
10. Congenital absence of pain sense (asymbolia) 1156	Principally metaphyses of long bones, although occasionally tubular bones of hands and feet and spine affected	Clinical features generally those of failure to respond to normal painful stimuli, including severe biting of tongue and lips. Fingers of child often badly self-bitten and mutilated. Corneal opacities caused by introduction of foreign bodies into eyes. Localised swelling, heat and redness around joints. Total absence or marked diminution of sense of pain	Four broad groups of radiological findings: gross fractures; stress fractures; osteomyelitis and suppurative arthritis; and neuropathic lesions around joints. Neuropathic lesions similar to those observed in tabes, syringomyelia, etc. Follow trauma	May resemble traumatised or 'battered' child syndrome. No definite aetiological factor. No specific neurological signs except diminution of sense of pain

TABLE IIB. *Other Traumatic Lesions of the Skeleton* (*contd.*)

Sub-group	Sites of Predilection	Special Features of Interest	Complications	Remarks
11. Traumatic lesions in children—acute, stress and chronic recurrent	*'Greenstick' fractures*; 50% in arm and forearm 20% in leg, **280**	Considered incomplete but both cortices involved. Remodelling can correct severe deformities, but not rotation. Long bone fractures common. Joint injuries unusual	Synostosis of radius and ulna. Femoral neck fractures have poor prognosis as post-traumatic necrosis of femoral head common	
	Fracture-separations of epiphyses, **280**	Usually also separate adjacent portion of metaphysis	Danger of premature epiphyseal fusion, especially important in lower limb	Hyperaemia may cause epiphyseal overgrowth, also chronic stress as in 'Little-Leaguer's Elbow'—large head of radius
	Epiphysiolysis (slipped epiphysis; adolescent coxa vara), **294**	Essentially a stress-type fracture-separation. Common in boys 10-15 years. Accentuated by obesity. Abnormal medial and posterior tilt femoral head with evidence metaphyseal remodelling	Complete reduction difficult. Post-traumatic necrosis of femoral head sometimes. Secondary degenerative joint disease relatively early in adult life	Commonly causes pain in knee of weeks or months duration. Minor forms believed to be responsible for degenerative joint disease, especially in males, later in life. Blount's disease (congenital tibia vara) essentially a stress disturbance of normal tibial epiphyses
	Traumatised child syndrome of Caffey, **281** (contrast with infantile cortical hyperostosis (also of Caffey) (see Table VIII)	Multiple injuries in young infants, with history concealed. 'Battered' baby syndrome. Fractures with hyperplastic callus and epiphyseal separations. Metaphyseal abnormalities (infraction, fragmentation or avulsion fractures) and periosteal reaction important features. Gross diaphyseal fractures not uncommon. Frequently associated with subdural haematomata and visceral injuries	With proper care and protection complications may be avoided and correction of deformities may take place by remodelling	Important medico-legally to demonstrate consecutive injuries in varying stages of repair
12. Degenerative joint disease (Appendicular) skeleton 'osteoarthritis, osteoarthrosis', **318**	*Post-traumatic.* Mainly affects joints subjected to chronic stress, especially if site of mechanical derangement, e.g. spine, hip, knee, ankle, 1st metatarsophalangeal joint, interphalangeal joints of hand, first toe	Joint space narrowing, eburnation joint surfaces, subchondral sclerosis, reactive bone formation, osteophytes (essentially protective to reduce mobility or avoid subluxation of affected joint), loose bodies	Hip lesions usually secondary to minimal epiphysiolysis in males, acetabular dysplasia in females and rheumatoid arthritis. Hallux valgus usual cause in feet	Osteophytes around interphalangeal joints result in Heberden's nodes. Pain-relieving therapy liable to permit excessive use of joints, especially hip and knee and may produce changes comparable to neuropathic disorder.
13. Vibration syndrome ('Driller's disease'), **1064**	Wrist and hand	Occupational disorder affecting users of compressed air drill (also metal grinders and chain-saw operators) for at least five to ten years. Holding hand especially affected	Symptoms consist of blanching, numbness and loss of fine sensation, reminiscent of Raynaud's phenomenon. Radiological features—post-traumatic subchondral cysts—often with evidence of degenerative joint disease	Arteriographic studies have demonstrated diminution of vascular supply to fingers, suggesting Raynaud's disease or scleroderma
14. Chondromalacia patellae, **306**	Articular cartilage of medial facet of patella	Predilection for males in second to fourth decade. Pain in region of patella with suspicion of locking. Presence of bony ridge of medial and less often lateral condyle of femur. Chronic stress may be causative factor. Pathologically, degenerative changes of articular cartilage of patella on medial aspect with fissures and ulcerations. Radiological findings positive in only 20%—include multiple, cystic, subarticular areas in patella. Best defined in axial views and with tomography	Secondary degenerative joint disease with joint space narrowing, osteophyte formation and synovitis. Juxta-articular osteoporosis not uncommon	Radiological studies often disappointing
15. Degenerative changes secondary to inflammatory arthritis, **814**	Secondary to pre-existing joint disorders, especially rheumatoid arthritis. Common in non-weight bearing joints	*Common features*. Joint space narrowing, relatively little reactive bone formation, relative absence of osteophytes. Examination of hands and feet may reveal old rheumatoid erosions	Hip lesions associated with medial migration of femoral head and protrusio acetabuli	Degenerative joint disease secondary to inflammatory arthritis comprises approximately 15% of primary or idiopathic 'osteoarthritis' cases
16. Degenerative disease of spine, **371**	Cervical and lumbar spine. Articulations between vertebral bodies and apophyseal joints. Referred to as 'spondylosis' when intervertebral discs are involved and 'osteoarthritis' when small joints affected. In cervical area degenerative changes common at C5-C6 and C6-C7 levels, particularly in elderly. Lower lumbar and lumbosacral areas commonly affected.	Narrowing of intervertebral spaces accompanied by osteophyte formation, often encroaching on related exit foramina, producing associated symptoms and signs; is common sequel to intervertebral disc derangement. True size of osteophytes incompletely revealed because of radiolucent cartilage caps	Entity indistinguishable clinically and even on plain films from herniated disc. Osteophytes may develop with degenerative changes posterior small joints, accentuating symptoms. Less likely thoracic and lumbar areas because of larger exit foramina	Osteophytes represent protective physiological response to disordered joint mechanism
17. Juvenile discogenic disorder (juvenile osteochondrosis—Scheuermann's disease), **360**	Thoracic spine—although any area of vertebral column may be affected. Children, adolescents, and young adults, most commonly affected. Males more than females. Common age incidence from 11 to 18 years.	Aetiology may lie in traumatic damage to articular plates, permitting herniation nucleus pulposus into vertebral bodies, with secondary vertebral irregularity and even partial destruction. Disc spaces invariably narrowed. Anterior third of vertebral body diminished in height	May result in secondary spondylosis. Residual 'limbus vertebra' (due to disc herniation) or ossicles may persist. Often produces severe kyphosis	'Ring' epiphyses may be fragmented. Disorder self-limiting. Many individuals affected may be asymptomatic. Often misdiagnosed as fracture or infective spondylitis

TABLE IIB. *Other Traumatic Lesions of the Skeleton (contd.)*

Sub-group	Sites of Predilection	Special Features of Interest	Complications	Remarks
18. Intervertebral disc derangements, 364	Lumbosacral and L4-L5 disc sites most frequently affected. Thoracic area relatively exempt. Cervical spine also frequently involved, particularly C5-C6 and C6-C7 levels	Radiological examination early in acute stage may be unrewarding, although suspicion may be aroused by mal-alignment of vertebral bodies. Scoliosis may be evident. Limitation of motion in flexion and extension views associated with muscle spasm. In later stages frank narrowing of intervertebral disc spaces evident. Instability then demonstrated. Traction spurs at affected level may be observed. Associated with chronic stress changes at attachments of anterior common ligaments	Degenerative changes may supervene, with formation of reactive osteophytes which represent attempt to limit movement at site of derangement	Myelography an important procedure to determine presence or absence of herniated discs
19. Spinal canal stenosis (underlying cause developmental), 375	Generally involves lumbar spinal canal although cervical spinal canal may be similarly affected. Usually in middle-aged and elderly individuals with definite predilection for males	Diagnosis may be made on plain films on A-P diameter of lumbar spine canal of less than 15 millimetres in lateral film and interpedicular distance AP films less than 25 millimetres. Vertebral bodies, pedicles and transverse processes frequently grossly enlarged. Myelographic studies often show multiple disc protrusions or even prominent dorsal defects without actual disc herniation. Opaque column narrowed. Complete obstruction may be encountered. Tortuous nerve roots simulating arteriovenous malformation may be evident	Failure to appreciate significance of syndrome may result in catastrophe, because more extensive surgical measures are required than in ordinary herniated disc	Syndrome results when inadequate development of spinal canal leads to failure of accommodation of nerve roots, dural membranes and extradural supporting tissues

TABLE III. *Infective Lesions*

Disorder	Organism	Sites of Predilection	Clinical Features	Pathological Findings	Radiological Features	Remarks
BACTERIAL DISEASES **Pyogenic osteomyelitis**, *Appendicular skeleton*, **392**	Varies. *Staph. strep.. Klebsiella, pseudomonas, col-iform bacilli, Salmonella*, etc.	Metaphyseal ends of bone around major joints: knee, hip, wrist. Fingers common site. Feet in diabetics. Involvement shafts of long bones not uncommon	Fever, swelling, tenderness, localised pain. Early symptoms and signs precede radiological abnormalities	Metaphysitis with bone destruction and abscess formation, periostitis, bone destruction and frank necrosis (sequestrum), involucrum formation	Usually haematogenous with metaphyseal involvement; early periosteal reaction. *diffuse* soft tissue swelling, sequestrum formation, lytic areas, involucrum, cortical and endosteal thickening. Brodie's abscess chronic stage	Radiological features influenced by antibiotics Klebsiella and salmonella infections tend to involve diaphysis of long bones Pseudomonas infections now commonly observed in narcotic addicts Epiphyseal plate usually a barrier to extension, after age of one year
Pyogenic osteomyelitis, *Axial skeleton*, **392**	As above	Lumbar spine commonest. Thoracic and cervical spine less common. Pelvis and skull occasionally	Fever, pain, tenderness, neurological deficits varying degrees	Bone destruction, abscesses, bone necrosis infrequently, new bone formation, relatively small paraspinal soft tissue inflammatory masses. Intervertebral discs invaded by inflammatory lesions frequently and relatively early	Erosive, lytic areas usually vertebral body. Reactive new bone common. Disc space narrowing frequent with adjacent vertebrae involved. Paraspinal masses less prominent than with tuberculosis. Calcification extremely rare. Osteoporosis unusual. Obvious sequestra infrequently observed. Serial studies show evolution and healing to be more rapid than in tuberculosis. Lesions usually solitary	Frequently associated with urinary tract infection, also 'mainliner' drug addicts. Difficult to differentiate from tuberculosis on single examination. Block on myelography rare
Infective discitis, **406**	Varies. Staphylococcus most common. Also *E. coli, proteus, salmonella*, etc.	Thoracic and lumbar areas	Generally affects adult males. Localised pain in back with symptoms and signs of preceding infection apparently controlled by antibiotic therapy, with resultant delay in presentation	Inflammatory granulation tissue generally replaces infected disc without formation of abscess. Granulation tissue extends into neural canal. Fibroblastic sequelae. Adjacent articular cartilages eroded, but subchondral plates generally intact, with reactive thickening of trabeculae	Initial abnormality narrowing of affected disc space with subsequent reactive sclerosis in adjacent portions of vertebral bodies. Articular erosions and bony prominences around disc space with buttressing may occur. Bony spurs fuse and infection becomes quiescent ultimately	Represents chronic, low-grade, smouldering infection. Frank osteomyelitis may occasionally develop with large concave erosions on each side of intervertebral space. Occurs occasionally in disc site with has undergone previous derangement—'*locus minoris resistentia*'

TABLE III. *Infective Lesions (contd.)*

Disorder	Organism	Sites of Predilection	Clinical Features	Pathological Findings	Radiological Features	Remarks
Pyogenic arthritis (pyarthrosis), 408	Mainly caused by *Staph. aureus*, but other organisms may be responsible, e.g. *pneumococcus*	Major peripheral joints (especially hip and knee) and small joints of hands and feet. Articular lesions much less common than purely osseous foci	Usually evidence of severe localised infection with systemic symptoms and signs and arthritic manifestations. Local pain, tenderness and swelling, fever, leucocytosis, increased sedimentation rate. Culture and identification of organism from joint diagnostic	May be secondary to systemic infection. Articular cartilage destroyed early, rapidly becoming necrotic and undergoing resorption by proteolytic enzymes. Infected granulation tissue may involve synovium and invade subchondral bone with early bone destruction. Osteoporosis subchondral area marked, but very little observed distal from joint. Granulation tissue formed. Often followed by fibrous and bony ankylosis	Soft tissue swelling, synovial effusion and synovitis. Localised bone atrophy and rapid appearance joint space narrowing. Localised subchondral bone erosions, hazy outline articular surfaces. Fibrous and even bony ankylosis later stages if cartilage entirely destroyed. Sequestrum formation sometimes observed. Obliteration of subchondral cortical white line an important radiological sign	Secondary subluxations occur, as in hips of infants. Atlanto-axial and other cervical spine subluxations may be associated with throat infections of children due to adjacent hyperaemia without actual joint infection
Tuberculosis *Appendicular skeleton,* **414**	*Tubercle bacillus* Usually haematogenous Human form common Also bovine form if milk not pasteurised Avian form very rare	Major joints most commonly. Hip, knee, ankle, wrist, elbow. Bones of hands and feet may be affected—dactylitis. Joint involvement much more common than purely osseous foci (compare pyogenic infections)	Low grade, indolent clinical history. Mild fever, low grade swelling, pain. Often associated with pulmonary tuberculosis. High correlation with renal tuberculosis	Tuberculous granulation tissue produces synovitis with erosion articular cartilages and invasion of subchondral bone. Caseation necrosis frequent, but gross sequestration uncommon. Marked osteoporosis. Reactive new bone infrequent	Synovitis common. Phemister triad—slow destruction of cartilage, peripheral articular defects and marked osteoporosis. Sequestra not uncommon, but small. Fibrous ankylosis may occur; bony ankylosis less common without secondary pyogenic infection. Reactive new bone slight. Draining sinuses common weight-bearing joints. Epiphyseal plate usually penetrated early as offers no barrier to extension	*Cystic tuberculosis* an infrequent variant—mostly in childhood—causing symmetrical osseous foci
Tuberculosis *Axial skeleton,* **414**	As above	Thoraco-lumbar area most common. Cervical spine relatively infrequent. S.I. joints frequently affected with spine involvement, usually unilateral. Flat bones not uncommon, pelvis, ribs, skull	Fever, back pain, neurological deficits may occur with paraplegia. Unusually bizarre forms may be observed in coloured races. Symptoms and signs usually milder and course more prolonged than in pyogenic infections	Tuberculous foci start usually anterior third vertebral body. Granulation tissue traverses paraspinal ligamentous areas invading disc cartilage with secondary compromise blood supply. Chiefly destructive lesions, but secondary new	Early changes—erosive lesions anterior third vertebral body ('gouge' defect) with extension remainder vertebrae causes disc narrowing. Spinal appendages may be affected initially with block on myelography. Destructive lesions cervical spine. (Quarter of lumbar and thoracic spine lesions stimulate reactive bone formation.) Paraspinal masses.	'Gouge' defect often attributable to aortic pulsation transmitted through paraspinal abscess. Multiple sites of skeletal involvement common. *Subligamentous spinal tuberculosis* may cause massive paravertebral abscesses with relatively little bone destruction. May mimic pyogenic osteomyelitis.

				bone formation common	either granulation tissue or pus, the rule. Eventually calcify. 'Gibbus' frequent. Sequestra occasionally observed—usually small. Sacro-iliac involvement usually unilateral
Anonymous atypical mycobacterial infection, 1138	Atypical mycobacteria—four groups: I, photochromogens; II, scotochromogens; III, nonchromogens; and IV, rapid growers	Generally diametaphyses and metaphyses of long bones, although any part of skeleton may be affected	Virtually similar to those of tuberculosis although tending to be milder	Similar to those described in tuberculosis—granulomatous disorder, usually without caseation	Skeletal involvement infrequent. Generally small, multiple, discrete lytic lesions with sclerotic borders and narrow zones of transition affecting metaphyses and diametaphyses of long bones. May simulate cystic tuberculosis. Spondylitis very rare	Lungs most commonly affected. Usual manifestations generally those of thin-walled cavities of upper lobes. Disorder more benign than classical tuberculosis
Brucellosis, 474	Three different members of genus *Brucella—melitensis, abortus* and *suis*	Axial skeleton most commonly, but lesions in areas major joints of appendicular skeleton—hips, knees, wrists—not uncommon	Transmitted by milk from affected animals, thus mainly found in countries where milk is not pasteurised. Clinical features indefinite. Low grade pyrexia, malaise and pain. 'Undulant' fever inconstant finding. Formerly endemic in Malta. Bacterial and serological tests available and confirmatory	Infection spreads usually from skin to lymph nodes, producing granulomatous reaction with necrosis. Organisms reach blood stream to disseminate reticuloendothelial tissues. Multiple small granulomata form, best studied bone marrow, liver and spleen. In bone locally destructive, but reactive new bone may form. Synovium of joints may be involved by granulomata with secondary cartilage destruction and subchondral bone erosions	In *spine* may simulate pyogenic or tuberculous infections. Paraspinal masses less frequent than in tuberculosis and do not calcify. Ultimately dense sclerosis with osteophytes and bony fusion common. In *appendicular* skeleton lesions may simulate tuberculous involvement with synovitis, articular erosion, joint space narrowing. Osteoporosis less common manifestation than in tuberculosis	May be indistinguishable radiologically from pyogenic and tuberculous lesions, pattern of changes being intermediate. Skeletal involvement occurs as a relatively late complication of the infection

r

TABLE III. *Infective Lesions (contd.)*

Disorder	Organism	Sites of Predilection	Clinical Features	Pathological Findings	Radiological Features	Remarks
Congenital syphilis, 444	*Treponema pallidum*	Major limb bones principally affected	Varies. Foetus may be dead at birth or only mild irritability with failure to thrive. Usually fever, bone pain and other signs and symptoms of generalised infection. Skin lesions, jaundice, hepato-splenomegaly, painful limbs (pseudoparalysis of Parrot). Positive serological tests	Syphilitic granulation tissue invades metaphyses in initial stages (metaphysitis or osteochondritis) disturbing growth process. Inflammatory periostitis subsequently followed in some instances by invasion cortex and spongiosa by granulation tissue with bone destruction	Three stages: (1) *Osteochondritis,* irregular erosive lesions metaphyses of long bones with fragmentation mainly knees, knees, shoulders and wrists (erosive lesions medial side of proximal tibial metaphysis—Wimberger zones). (2) *Periostitis*—usually diffuse, widespread, symmetrical and affecting long bones occurs several months later. 'Bone within a bone' effect as cortical thickening occurs. (3) *Osteitis.* Later still. 1st and 2nd years. Relatively uncommon. Simulates lesions of pyogenic osteomyelitis with destruction cortex and spongiosa, but lytic areas tend to be fusiform. No sequestra generally	Three stages need not follow in orderly fashion. Several stages may co-exist. Adequate treatment specific. Other late changes include 'sabre shin', hydrarthrosis knee. Infantile lesions may recur in adolescence Positive serological determination generally but not invariably present. Late skeletal manifestations usually observed in latter part of first or second decades of life. Periosteal reaction with new bone formation of proximal two-thirds of tibia late effect. Other late features include gummata and arthritic changes due to recurrent metaphysitis. Clutton's joint without associated bone destruction may be present. Hutchinson's teeth may develop.
Acquired syphilis, 450	*Treponema pallidum*	Any part of skeleton may be affected, but limb bones— mainly femur, tibia and radius—and calvarium, clavicle and pelvis commonly involved. Lesions unifocal or disseminated More superficial portions of skeleton frequently involved—skull, clavicle and tibia	Late manifestation usually of acquired disease occurring mostly middle-aged and elderly. Localised bone pain common. Skeletal deformity may occur if considerable new bone formation develops	Periostitis may occur secondary stage with lymphocytes, plasma cells and leukocytes. In tertiary stage bone destruction by diffuse process or gummata (areas caseation necrosis surrounded by inflammatory reaction with vascular proliferation and perivascular infiltrate)	Combination of bone destruction and new bone formation most frequent, but purely lytic or blastic lesions may be encountered. Periosteal reaction not uncommon. Gumma may produce localised destructive lesion simulating neoplasm. Sequestra rare. 'Sabre shin', particularly bilateral, practically diagnostic. Reactive new bone common. Small sequestra may be present, but unusual to detect radiologically	Neuropathic skeletal disease late manifestation of acquired syphilis, but not actually associated with syphilitic inflammatory lesions (see Table II). Serological studies usually positive, but skeletal manifestations of acquired tertiary syphilis may be encountered with consistently negative serological results
Yaws, 458	*Treponema pertenue*	Tubular bones of hands and feet, long bones, pelvis, skull and facial bones	Generally acquired late first decade, mainly confined to tropics	Tertiary lesions similar pathologically to syphilis	Three stages simulate syphilis although far less distinct. Lucent defects of cortex and spongiosa, florid periosteal reactions, reactive new bone in medullary cavities, particularly late, considerable osteoporosis with secondary bowing limb bones. 'Sabre shin' as in syphilis. Extensive joint deformities with consequent bony ankylosis	Differential diagnosis from syphilis may be impossible radiologically, clinically and even by serological methods Two points of distinction from syphilis exist in radiological features. Metaphysitis of congenital syphilis does not occur in yaws in infants and children and dactylitis in yaws considerably more common than in syphilis

	Radius, ulna and tibia most commonly affected in tertiary phase. Destructive lesions of maxilla may occur, producing bulbous enlargement known as *goundou*. Spontaneous resolution may occur in all three stages	Initial infection generally extragenital and through direct contact. Skin ulceration particularly of face, limbs, plantar aspects of feet, painful bony and soft tissue masses, arthralgia, soft tissue and joint contractures. Accompanying malnutrition and osteomalacia common in endemic areas	Radiological diagnosis may be suggested by evidence of neuropathic disease of hands and feet although such changes may be indistinguishable from other causes of neuropathic lesions. Calcification in large peripheral nerve diagnostic but uncommon Destructive lesions may occasionally involve skeletal sites other than hands and feet—nasal bones, nasal spine of maxilla and bones of leg, including patella.
Leprosy, 468 *Mycobacterium leprae* (*Hansen's bacillus*)	Major joints of extremities with predilection for hands and feet. Nose and maxilla may be involved	Skin lesions in *tuberculoid* form consist of epithelial cells in clusters forming granulomatous masses. Early destruction of nerves in dermis. Leprae bacilli sparse in tissues. *Leproid* form —marked proliferation of histiocytes in superficial layers of skin with invasion of nerve fibres and blood vessel walls. Caseous abscesses may develop around nerves. Leprae bacilli very common in tissue sections	Three groups of changes: 1. *Specific leprous bone changes* which occur in only about 15% of patients—*osteitis of leprosy*—with two subgroups: (a) *lepra-reactive group*—various types of bone destruction particularly of the hands, including dissolution of terminal tufts and destruction resulting in twisted fingers; (b) *leproma of bone*—represented by large nutrient foramina of phalanges of hand and cystlike lesions in distal end of a proximal phalanx 2. *Non-specific osteitis group*—observed in about 50% of patients. Skeletal changes usually in hands and feet, essentially neuropathic in type with or without infection. Frequently consist of terminal tuft erosions followed by absorption of entire phalanges. Superadded infection may hasten bone destruction. Absence of significant osteoporosis even in presence of infection 3. Another *non-specific group*—osteoporosis secondary to skin contractures, general debility, inadequate diet and old age may be observed in small percentage of cases
		Predilection for Asiatic and African countries with substandard hygiene. *Tuberculoid* form relatively mild with granulomatous, discrete skin nodules. *Lepromatous* type more malignant—widespread confluent skin lesions. Erythema nodosa common. Nerve involvement predominant feature, with secondary effects of loss of skin sensitivity, localised infections etc. Skin contractures and secondary infection common	

TABLE III. *Infective Lesions (contd.)*

Disorder	Organism	Sites of Predilection	Clinical Features	Pathological Findings	Radiological Features	Remarks
Tropical ulcer, 647	Usually but not invariably organisms of Vincent group. May be mixed variety of bacteria	Tibia and fibula	Peak incidence between 20 and 30 years of age, with no distinct sex predilection. Observed mainly in Central Africa. Lower limb bones involved—tibia more commonly. Recurrent chronic ulcers involving lower limb produce skin cicatrisation, deep pigmentation and lymphoedema. Bowing of long bones, flexion deformities of knee; other deformities of feet and ankles may be associated in later stages	Related mainly to chronic infection of skin, subcutaneous tissues and bone. Inflammatory granulation tissue, abscess formation and sinus tracts with invasion of cortex and spongiosa with extensive sequestrum formation	In initial stage of development of superficial ulcer of leg; localised soft tissue swelling apparent. Periosteal reaction may result in fusiform or even 'sunburst' appearance suggesting malignant neoplasm. Cortical destruction and sequestration follow. With healing, thickened, sclerotic cortex results in classical 'ivory ulcer osteoma'. Expansion of medullary cavity may produce 'ulcer osteoma'	In approximately 2% of patients squamous cell carcinoma may develop in superficial area of ulceration. Radiological signs of this complication include increase in soft tissue swelling and loss of sharply defined outline of skeletal lesion, with increasing bone destruction. Exuberant periosteal reaction may be encountered
Histoplasmosis, 464	*Histoplasmosis capsulatum*	Skeletal lesions rare. Flat bones—pelvis, ribs, calvarium—and major long bones occasionally affected	Systemic disease very similar to tuberculosis in effect on lungs and mediastinum. Primary and secondary pulmonary forms, usually mild with infiltrate and lymph node involvement. Initially, respiratory infection. Dissemination infrequently	Histiocyte response initially in affected tissues. Subsequent histiocytic granulation with necrosis and caseation. Calcification common in healing stage, particularly in lungs and mediastinal lymph nodes. Similar lesions in skeleton in disseminated form. Intradermal and serological tests available	Infrequent instances of skeletal lesions (disseminated haematogenous) flat bones—calvarium, pelvis—may be affected. Also small tubular bones. Small, discrete lytic lesions may occur, although appearance may simulate pyogenic osteomyelitis	Skeletal lesions not diagnostic unless presence of disseminated disease established. Disease widespread many parts U.S.A. Sporadic cases anywhere. Contracted from soil, excreta chickens, birds (pigeons) and bats. Skeletal lesions very rare in histoplasmosis capsulatum form
	Histoplasmosis duboisii (African type)	Skeleton much more frequently involved than in capsulatum type. Lungs usually spared. Skin lesions common. Localised and disseminated forms. Tends to be self-limiting in localised form, but often	Often self-limiting disorder	Chronic infective process—histiocytes, lymphocytes, granulation tissue, necrosis and caseation	Irregular areas of bone destruction occasionally solitary, but usually multiple, often accompanied by periosteal reaction and reactive new bone formation. Paraspinal masses common in spinal involvement, with lytic lesions of vertebral bodies and relative preservation of intervertebral discs	Extensive lesions in long bones may simulate round cell neoplasms (e.g. Ewing's tumour). Generally, destructive lesions non-specific, suggesting infective aetiology

Disease	Causative organism	Bones/parts affected	Distribution and clinical features	Pathology	Radiological features
FUNGUS DISEASES, 478 **Mycetoma (Madura foot), 500**	*Madurella mycetome*; *Madura mycetes* and *actinomycetes* groups of moulds. Yellow and black spore types	Feet mainly affected, but other parts of skeleton occasionally involved. Fatal when visceral spread affects lymphatic system and liver. Spinal involvement with paraplegia may develop. Draining sinuses common	Prevalent in tropical areas with dry season and poor hygienic conditions affecting mainly bare-footed individuals. Found commonly parts of Africa, India, Mexico. Transmitted from soil through skin wound causing subcutaneous nodule and draining sinus of foot	Subcutaneous nodules and draining sinuses consisting of inflammatory granulation tissue, abscesses and cyst-like cavities. Muscle and bone secondarily invaded. Replacement fibrosis and reparative bone sclerosis common features. Secondary pyogenic infection often superimposed	Initially soft tissue nodule followed by soft tissue swelling plantar aspect of foot with obliteration soft tissue planes. Pressure erosions of adjacent bone, multiple lytic defects and sometimes widespread extensive destruction of bone with florid periosteal reaction and reactive new bone characteristic. Yellow spore types produce infiltrating type of skeletal lesions while encapsulated black spore types generally result in circumscribed bone defects. Lesions may simulate osteosarcoma because of excessive proliferative periosteal and cortical reaction. Bones other than feet may be affected raising question of haematogenous spread
Actinomycosis, 479	Actinomycosis Israeli generally and occasionally *Actinomycosis bovis*, which is ordinarily pathogenic for animals (actually bacterial). *Nocardioses* organisms may be responsible	Mandible, flat bones (pelvis, ribs), spine, major joints	World wide distribution. Not uncommon Southwestern U.S. and Central America. Rare Great Britain. Usually chronic affecting cervico-facial soft tissues, spine, lungs, pleura and G.I. tract (ileocaecal area). Draining sinuses common. Two major forms: *cervico-facial* and *abdominal*. Disease may generalise and prove fatal. Skeletal and joint lesions infrequent, may be painful	*Cervico-facial form.* Inflammatory lesions starting in mandible, frequently in tooth socket, and spreading to involve soft tissues angle of jaw and neck with abscess and draining sinus. Secondary spread to spine, ribs and other skeletal sites. *Abdominal form.* Begins in colon or appendix. Ulcerations in intestinal mucosa with abscesses containing yellow granules. Chronic granulomatous process with many giant cells. Skeletal lesions similar, resembling pyogenic infection	Frank destruction of a mottled permeating type the rule, occasionally with reactive new bone formation. Joint involvement mimics tuberculosis closely, but with less bone atrophy. *Rib:* infiltration with periosteal reaction may suggest neoplasm. Accompanying pleuritis and peripleuritis common. *Spine:* destructive lesions with relative preservation intervertebral disc spaces. Paravertebral abscesses tend to be smaller than in tuberculosis and do not calcify. Radiological features of an inflammatory rib lesion with pleuritis and peripleuritis or spine lesion simulating tuberculosis, but with intact intervertebral discs, frequently accompanied by draining sinuses, should suggest the diagnosis. Lesions in joints of appendicular skeleton may simulate tuberculosis

TABLE III. *Infective Lesions (contd.)*

Disorder	Organism	Sites of Predilection	Clinical Features	Pathological Findings	Radiological Features	Remarks
Coccidioido-mycosis, 478	*Coccidioidis immitis*	Spine, pelvis, ribs, skull, long bones	Endemic S.W., part of U.S. particularly sections of California, Arizona, New Mexico. Also found in Mexico. Two main forms. *Pulmonary-mediastinal nodal lesions* (common). Generally benign with no skeletal involvement. Mimics primary tuberculosis. *Progressive disseminated form*. Simulates miliary tuberculosis with symptoms and signs of overwhelming infection. Pain common at site of skeletal lesions. Draining sinuses frequent. Skin test and serological tests available	In primary pulmonary form initially pneumonic consolidation in lung with involvement adjacent lymph nodes similar to primary tuberculous complex. Initial acute response to organism resembles pyogenic infections with spheroid cells which may contain endospores. Granulomatous lesions chronic stage contain histiocytes and giant cells. In progressive form caseous nodules and abscesses with numerous giant cells may invade multiple structures. Lesions may be suppurative or granulomatous	Predominantly destructive lesions with reactive new bone in chronic or healing phases. Metaphyses and diametaphyseal areas of long bones commonly involved. Sequestrum formation infrequent. Flat bone lesions tend to be discrete, but may be confluent and expanding. Bony prominences most commonly affected. Characteristic destructive lesions observed in vertebral bodies with extensive paraspinal abscesses simulating tuberculosis. Intervertebral disc spaces frequently escape involvement in contrast with tuberculosis. Actual joint involvement in appendicular skeleton infrequently encountered in contrast to tuberculosis	Draining sinuses common, particularly from spine and ribs. Skeletal lesions particularly prone to dissemination in coloured races, with increased severity of disease
Blastomycosis (North American form), **484** S. American form also exists	*Blastomyces dermatitidis* (North American form) *Paracoccidioides* (South American form)	Limb bones, pelvis, spine. No part of skeleton immune	North American form common Southern and Southeastern U.S.: South American form in Brazil, Columbia, Central America. Both types practically unknown in Great Britain. In N.A. form infection may start in lungs (by inhalation) with pneumonia. Also cutaneous origin with skin abscesses and draining sinuses. Haematogenous spread to skeleton from either pulmonary or cutaneous origins, or skeleton may be affected by contiguous spread from skin lesions.	Characteristic tissue response in most areas involved combination suppurative and epithelioid cells with numerous giant cells. Particularly true in skeletal lesions. Bone necrosis frequent. Micro-abscesses common in skin and subcutaneous tissues	Skeletal lesions virtually always frankly and grossly destructive with sequestrum formation common. Simulate severe fulminating pyogenic osteomyelitis. New bone formation extremely rare. Metaphyseal predilection in long bones	Frankly destructive aggressive skeletal lesions which appear infective in presence of draining sinuses, particularly in an endemic area, should suggest the diagnosis

	Organism	Bones affected	Clinical features	Pathology	Radiology
			Pain and draining sinuses at site of skeletal lesions. Joint involvement rare in contrast to actinomycosis, but septic arthritis may occur. Skeletal lesions similar in both forms. Skin test available		Skeletal findings not diagnostic. Often associated with pulmonary disease. May be complication of prolonged corticosteroid therapy
Torulosis (cryptococosis), 484	*Torula histolytica* (cryptococcus neoformans)	Flat bones (mainly pelvis) and major long bones. Short tubular bones infrequently	Chronic systemic fungus disease found throughout world. Frequently fatal outcome, particularly with meningeal involvement. Being observed with increasing frequency, particularly in patients treated with corticosteroids, as secondary invader in chronic lymphoproliferative disease. Mainly affects lungs and central nervous system. Skeletal lesions rare—usually haematogeneous. Features depend on extent and severity of disease	Paucity of cellular reaction with characteristic absence suppuration, necrosis or caseation. On occasion, chronic inflammatory response with giant cells and fibrous tissue. Organism may produce gelatinous masses in lungs and small cysts in brain	Skeletal lesions practically always lytic. Usually discrete lucent defects. Periosteal reaction common in lesions of long bones. Bone sclerosis very rare

TABLE III. *Infective Lesions (contd.)*

Disorder	Organism	Sites of Predilection	Clinical Features	Pathological Findings	Radiological Features	Remarks
PARASITIC DIS-EASES INVOLV-ING SKELETON **Hydatid disease (echinococ-cosis), 490**	*Taenia echinococ-cus.* Definitive host—dog, wolf. Intermediate host—sheep, cattle, dogs or man	Pelvis and spine main-ly but limb bones occasionally affected	Endemic in sheep-farming areas. Has been observed in Australasia, many parts Asian continent, Middle East, S. America, Iceland, N. Can-ada, Wales. Dis-ease in man usually acquired from sheep-dog. Cysts ultimately develop from larvae. About 75% trap-ped in liver, 15% in lungs. Remainder settle in any body structure, including skeleton. 25% of those affected, asymptomatic. Bone lesions 2% of cases. Slowly progressive dis-ease. Allergic manifestations common—urticaria and angioneurotic oedema. Eosino-philia common. Rupture of cysts—particularly in lung and peritoneal cavity—may pro-mote anaphylactic shock. Skeletal le-sions generally, but not invariably, symptomatic. Localised pain common. Com-plement fixation and intradermal skin test important diagnostic aids	Cysts consist of outer laminated and inner germinal layer containing clear fluid. Daugh-ter cysts develop within cysts. Cysts may collapse, un-dergoing fibrosis and calcification. May become secon-darily infected with suppuration. Rup-ture of cysts and re-lease of fluid mainly responsible for al-lergic manifesta-tions and eosino-philia. Rupture into peritoneal and pleural cavities may initiate inflammat-ory changes, par-ticularly if cysts infected	Skeletal changes brought about by pressure in medullary cav-ity from multiple daughter cysts. Ill-defined defects ini-tially followed by more sharply defined lytic lesions with sclerotic border. Cysts areas may become expanding and confluent with loss of normal bone architecture. Cortex may be perforated with rupture into soft tissues, secondary endocyst forma-tion and calcification. Slow spread through entirety of affected bone. Disease may spread across joints	Expanding skeletal lesions may simulate neoplasm because of extensive destruction. Supporting evidence may be provided by cysts in lung or in liver. Ectocyst frequently calcifies in liver, but not in lung
Ainhum, 462	Unknown (? parasite)	Fifth toe, but other toes may be involved	More common in Af-rican males. Usu-ally 4th to 5th de-cades of life. Fis-sure on plantar sur-face affected toe with skin hyper-trophy, followed by oedema and con-stricting band.	Soft tissue groove generally beginning on medial aspect of involved fifth toe with fibrosis of ad-jacent dermis and formation of hyper-keratotic band within epidermis. Pressure atrophy of	Soft tissue constriction with bone absorption and marked tapering of phalanges of affected digit. Ultimately loss of involved phalanges	Mainly observed in blacks liv-ing in warm climates, par-ticularly in West Africa, but sporadic cases encountered in Southern part of United States, virtually always in black race

Melioidosis, 463	*Pfeifferella whitmori*	Any portion of skeleton, lungs, gastrointestinal tract commonly affected. Sepsis not infrequent in fulminating cases, which may terminate fatally within few days	May be painless early. Secondary infection may occur. Autoamputation often end-result underlying bone causes tapering effect—spontaneous amputation	In acute stages aggregates of abscesses with polymorphonuclear leukocytes, necrotic debris with giant cells and haemosiderin. In chronic stages chronic abscesses consisting of central area of necrosis with mononuclear cells and granulation tissue	Disseminated destructive lesions, characteristic of chronic inflammation, but non-specific in type	Skeletal involvement rare. Diagnosis must be suspected when unexplained suppurative lesions with pulmonary involvement and discharging sinuses are encountered in patients who have been exposed to the disease in endemic area
Neonatal transplacental rubella syndrome, 1132	Rubella virus	Metaphyses of major long bones	Mental deficiency, dwarfism, cataracts, thrombocytopenic purpura, hepatosplenomegaly, congenital cardiovascular lesions	May be due to metabolic and nutritional trophic disturbances rather than infective osteomyelitis caused by rubella virus. Histological sections rarely obtained. Excessive fibrosis and deficient ossification described in one specimen from rib	Observed in at least half the infants with this syndrome. Metaphyseal irregularities particularly around the knee; lucent horizontal metaphyseal bands and alternating vertical bands of sclerosis and translucency. 'Celery stalk' appearance of metaphyses	Rubella in pregnant mother in first trimester most dangerous period. Osseous changes usually regress slowly and most often completely over a course of several weeks
Chronic granulomatous disease of childhood (Landing-Shirkey syndrome), 1124	Varies. Usually of low-grade virulence. Generally *Staphylococcus aureus*, *Staphylococcus epidermidis*, *Serratio maricascens*	Any portion of skeleton; tubular bones of hands and feet most often affected. Other areas besides skeleton involved, e.g. lungs, liver, gastrointestinal tract, genitourinary tract, spleen, pericardium and brain	Principally affects male children. Transmitted as X-linked recessive. Usually history of protracted febrile illnesses in a child with recurrent infections throughout infancy and early childhood. Eczematoid and purulent skin lesions, adenitis, protracted pneumonia and pulmonary and cerebral abscesses common. Manifestations of typical osteomyelitis may be absent since organisms generally of low-grade violence	Disorder due to functional defect in polymorphonuclear leukocytes with inability to destroy bacteria. *In vitro* tests show deficiency of intercellular killing capacity of bacteria by leukocytes. Relatively simple diagnostic procedure is quantitative nitro blue tetrazolium test (NBT) in which granulocytes lack ability to reduce NBT to blue formazone. Osteomyelitic foci no different than in simple osteomyelitis	Generally extensive destruction at site of osteomyelitic focus, with very little sclerosis observed in healing phase. Tubular bones of hands and feet often affected. May often simulate tuberculous dactylitis because of excessive granulomatous response. Other radiological findings depend on organ or areas involved. May simulate eosinophil granuloma	Antibiotic therapy unsuccessful unless given continuously and over long period of time. Residual stigmata of osteomyelitis of affected bone generally minimal and virtually absent if adequately treated. Film of abdomen may be diagnostic because of multiple, small, focal calcifications in liver due to healed abscesses

TABLE IV. *Classification of Bone Tumours and Tumour-like Lesions.*
(modified from the classification of the Royal National Orthopaedic Hospital, London, 1969)

IA. *Presumed to arise from skeletal connective tissue—forming BONE*

	Tumour	Age of Incidence in Decades	Sex Incidence M F	Sites of Predilection	Clinical Features	Pathological Findings	Radiological Features	Remarks
Benign	**Osteoma, 568**	**345**	1 : 1	Virtually always arise in membranous bone, particularly skull and paranasal sinuses. Very rare in long bones. Virtually all lesions called osteomata arising from appendicular skeleton represent osteochondromata	Absent or due to pressure. Often incidental finding in paranasal sinuses. Rarely, cribriform plate may be eroded to produce pneumocephalus	Solid mass compact or cancellous new bone generally originating in membranous bone of calvarium from outer table or paranasal sinuses	Spheroid, well-circumscribed and dense, bony masses generally less than 1 cm in diameter. Lesions in skull may simulate meningiomata	Virtually no instance of malignant transformation. May be associated with polyposis of colon—Gardner's syndrome—in which true osteomata of appendicular skeleton may occur, as well as osteomata of skull. Fibrous osteoma in children may resemble true osteoma, but are probably variants of fibrous dysplasia
	Osteoid osteoma, 538	**123 4**	2 : 1	Two-thirds affect appendicular skeleton, especially proximal and distal segments of femur and proximal half of tibia. Much less common in axial skeleton	Localised pain of weeks or months, worse at night, relieved by aspirin. Exceptionally, marked weakness, associated muscular atrophy of affected limb. Scoliosis in spinal lesions	Small focus osteoblasts initially replaced by osteoid or fibrous tissue (nidus). Usually considerable reactive new bone in periphery which is highly vascular. Especially prominent with parosteal location, early age and long duration, but minimal around intracapsular and medullary lesions. Central nidus varies from 0·5 to 2·0 cm in diameter	Round or oval area of translucency containing dense nidus less than 2 cm in diameter. Extent of sclerotic zone increases with age of lesion, youth of patient and peripheral location in bone. Overlying periosteal reaction may occur. Tendency to considerable sclerosis in younger children. Affected long bone in children may increase in length In spine, area of sclerosis generally in neural arch, producing scoliosis with convexity to opposite side	Some medullary lesions very elusive. Tomography required. Differentiation from chronic osteomyelitis important, which may be established by angiography demonstrating 'blush' in venous phase in contrast to Brodie's abscess

Benign	**Benign osteo-blastoma, 543**	1 23.4	1 : 1	Over half occur in spine and occasionally flat bones. Predilection for neural arches although lesions occasionally observed in vertebral body. Remainder affect long bones and short tubular bones	Localised pain and tenderness at site of lesion is usual complaint. Pain generally less severe than in osteoid osteoma without relief by aspirin. Neurological deficits and even paraplegia from spinal lesion may occur	Haemorrhagic, irregular, relatively large mass of osteoid comprises nidus from 2 to 10 cm. Frequently confused with osteoid osteoma histologically or even osteosarcoma	*Axial Skeleton.* Tend to be bone forming, although radiolucent nidus usually present. Neural arch mainly affected, although vertebral body may be involved. *Appendicular Skeleton.* Lesions mainly osteolytic, although long standing long neoplasms may provoke intense reactive sclerosis. Lesion often elongated in long bone but tends to be more focal in short tubular bone. Interspersed areas of new bone formation and radiolucent zones commonly encountered	Radiological features in long bones may be extremely protean and bizarre. Because of relationship to osteoid osteoma histologically and occasionally radiologically term *osteoid osteoma—osteoblastoma complex* suggested. Controversy exists concerning possible transformation to osteosarcoma
Malignant	**Osteosar-coma, 592**	1 23	3 : 2	Appendicular skeleton most frequently involved—90%. At least half around knee. Any bone may be affected	Pain and swelling, often of only a few weeks duration. Low grade pyrexia. Hence clinical resemblance to acute osteomyelitis in many cases. Pathological fractures not uncommon cause of presentation	Presumed to arise from primitive fibrous tissue or osteoblasts. Extremely varied cellular pattern. Predominant tissue either malignant osteoid, bone, cartilage or fibrous tissue. Cellular spectrum varies from highly anaplastic, plump connective tissue cells with hyperchromatic nuclei to dense tumour bone with few stromal cells. Most lesions show considerable neoplastic osteoid. New bone frequently composed non-neoplastic osteocytes—response to tumour. Lesions often highly vascular	Neoplastic osteoid tissue radiolucent accounting for lytic defects with wide endosteal zone of transition and cortical destruction. New bone formation causes increasing irregular density. 'Codman triangles' of reactive periosteal bone. 'Sunburst' spiculation characteristic but relatively uncommon. Epiphyseal plate temporary barrier to spread. Soft tissue extensions common	Most common primary malignant bone tumour but may be simulated by bizarre infections and unusual traumatic lesions. 'Cannon ball' metastases to lungs may occur early and be bone-forming. May metastasise to pleura, producing calcification and ossification. *Multicentric osteosarcomatosis* a rare variant, with simultaneously-appearing blastic lesions often throughout skeleton

TABLE IV. *Classification of Bone Tumours and Tumour-like Lesions* (*contd.*)
(modified from the classification of the Royal National Orthopaedic Hospital, London, 1969)

IA. *Presumed to arise from skeletal connective tissue—forming* BONE (*contd.*)

	Tumour	Age of Incidence in Decades	Sex Incidence M F	Sites of Predilection	Clinical Features	Pathological Findings	Radiological Features	Remarks
Malignant	**Parosteal osteosarcoma (juxtacortical), 600**	2 34	2 : 3	Most often around metaphysis of long bones and particularly distal end of femur and proximal end of tibia. Proximal portion of humerus occasionally	Lesion may be asymptomatic for long periods. Pain generally mild and intermittent. Constitutional signs and symptoms generally absent	Vary considerably although degree of malignancy low in comparison with classical osteosarcoma. Lesion may have cartilaginous cap suggesting osteochondroma. Invasion of medulla by tumour generally indicates unfavourable prognosis and histological sections in such instances resemble osteosarcoma	Initially small foci new bone gradually growing and coalescing to become tumour mass around shaft of parent bone. In early stages neoplasm tends to be partially separated from bone of origin by narrow zone of flucency. Peripheral border usually lobulated. When tumour infiltrates cortex and medulla of parent bone, observe areas of lysis interspersed with new bone formation	Must be distinguished from posttraumatic mineralisation ('myositis ossificans'), in which bony lesion is more dense at periphery and less dense in central segment, in contrast to juxtacortical osteosarcoma in which opposite occurs
	Paget's sarcoma, 628	5 67 8	2 : 1	Femur most commonly involved followed, in order of frequency, by humerus, innominate bones, skull and tibia	Increasing pain and swelling at site of lesion. Soft tissue mass occasionally palpated. Approximately one-third of patients present with pathological fracture	Highly variable in appearance. At least half the cases predominantly osteosarcoma with fibrosarcoma not infrequent. Considered to be potentially a mixed mesodermal sarcoma, with varying types of mesenchymal malignant tissue. Even reticulum cell sarcoma, giant cell sarcoma and chondrosarcoma have been reported. All elements may be observed in same specimen	Approximately one quarter of cases bone forming, with pattern resembling osteosarcoma or chondrosarcoma. Three-quarters of lesions essentially lytic, which are either grossly expanding or may show permeating, destructive pattern	Occurs in less than 1% of cases of Paget's disease. Multicentric forms encountered rarely—may be both lytic and boneforming in same patient
	Sarcoma following irradiation, 634	67 8		Site of irradiation	Pain and swelling	Histological pattern usually of fibrosarcoma or osteosarcoma	Similar pattern to sarcomata arising *de novo*. Long latent period (up to 20 yrs). Always have received more than 3000 r.	Malignant change has been observed after irradiation of some benign tumours

			Site	Clinical features	Pathology	Radiology	Comments
Multicentric osteosarcoma, 1038	1 23 4		Metaphyses of long bones. Flat bones including innominate bones, thorax and skull commonly affected. Disseminated distribution	Usually those of rapidly developing, fatal disorder with pain at multiple skeletal sites. Markedly elevated alkaline phosphatase common	Similar to solitary osteosarcoma of bone-forming variety	Multicentric lesions virtually always osteoblastic and frequently numerous. Each lesion shows classical appearance of solitary osteosarcoma with florid, coarse, periosteal reaction and Codman triangles. Affected area usually intensely opaque. Cortex of long bone often penetrated by tumour, invading soft tissues. Cartilage plate may be traversed into ossification centre	Multiple lesions have been considered metastatic from primary focus, but authenticity of this entity now accepted Counterpart exists in Paget's disease with development of multicentric osteosarcomata. In latter malignant lesions either osteolytic or osteoblastic in contrast to multicentric osteosarcomatosis without Paget's disease in which lesions are essentially blastic

IB. *Presumed to arise from skeletal connective tissue—forming* CARTILAGE

			Site	Clinical features	Pathology	Radiology	Comments
Solitary enchondroma, 514	34 5	1 : 1	Hands, feet, long bones, flat bones. Usually diaphyseal or diametaphyseal location	Painless swelling. Often incidentally discovered. May fracture	Focus of cartilage cells which may undergo secondary calcification. In short tubular bones cartilage cells typically show solitary nuclei. Double and even triple nuclei present in enchondromata of long bones. Malignant potential for lesions in long bones and flat bones in contrast to short tubular bones of hands and feet	Medullary translucency with narrow zone of transition may expand and thin overlying cortex and produce subendosteal sclerosis with scalloping as well as thickening of cortex, particularly in long bones. Calcification within lesions frequent—punctate or circular densities	Lesions in long bones and flat bones liable to sarcomatous transformation in contrast to short tubular bones Must be distinguished from medullary infarct. Enchondroma is expansile in contrast to infarct. Fibro-osseous wall around infarct virtually never present in enchondroma Multiple enchondromata constitute dyschondroplasia (Ollier's disease)
Enchondromatosis, 104 (Ollier's disease)	See Table IB—Generalised Congenital Disorders						
Maffucci syndrome, 1074	See Table IB—Generalised Congenital Disorders						

Benign

TABLE IV. *Classification of Bone Tumours and Tumour-like Lesions* (*contd.*)
(modified from the classification of the Royal National Orthopaedic Hospital, London, 1969)

IB. *Presumed to arise from skeletal connective tissue—forming CARTILAGE* (*contd.*)

Tumour	Age of Incidence in Decades	Sex Incidence M F	Sites of Predilection	Clinical Features	Pathological Findings	Radiological Features	Remarks
Parosteal (juxtacortical) chondroma, 516	2 3 **4 5**	1 : 1	Tubular bones of hands and feet, major long bones and even flat bones—clavicle and rib	Pain and swelling in contrast to often painless solitary enchondroma	Similar to solitary enchondroma	Soft tissue mass characteristic. Observed to contain calcified deposits in at least half the cases, adjacent to smooth erosion of outer surface of cortex. Lesion may stimulate formation of sclerotic endosteal margin unlike usual enchondroma	Reactive new bone frequently encountered at medullary base of lesion Sufficient experience regarding potential of malignant transformation not yet acquired
Benign chondroblastoma, 548	*1* **2 3** *4*	2 : 1	Particular affinity for proximal ends of humerus, femur and tibia. Tubular bones and flat bones, particularly innominate bones, also involved	Low-grade pain, tenderness, and limitation of motion of adjacent joint	Consists of chondroid tissue containing polyhedral cells, giant cells, focal areas of calcification, collagenisation and, on occasion, areas of haemorrhage. Numerous giant cells may suggest giant cell tumour. Sometimes confused with chondromyxoid fibroma. Malignant metaplasia extremely rare	Lytic area generally originating in ossification centre of long bone in growing skeleton, although lesion may arise in an apophysis (e.g. trochanter of femur). Adjacent metaphysis may be involved as lesion crosses growth plate. Lesion usually well demarcated, spheroid or ovoid with narrow zone of transition. Generally short, focal and indolent. Endosteal scalloping often. Pathological fractures uncommon. Amorphous or spotty calcification observed in approximately half the mature tumours	Formerly regarded as atypical giant cell tumour Tumour may become considerably opaque in later stages due to extensive calcification and even suggestion of new bone formation

Benign

Chondromyx-oid fibroma, 554	1 23 4	1 : 1	Proximal end of tibia most often involved (diametaphysis). Proximal and distal ends of femur and short, tubular bones of hands and feet not infrequently affected	Localised pain and swelling, generally of long duration and generally more severe than in chondroblastoma	Lesion related to chondroblastoma. Contains cartilaginous elements, but fibrous and myxoid tissues often predominate. Calcified deposits in late stages	Destructive, expanding lesion tending to be eccentric. May provoke much reactive sclerosis. Narrow zone of transition usually, but occasionally wide enough to suggest malignancy. Endosteal sclerosis and cortical thickening frequent findings. Although matrix of tumour largely cartilaginous, flecks of calcification distinctly unusual radiologically. Lesion tends to be elongated and often aggressive in contrast to chondroblastoma	May encounter lesions in subarticular location of a long bone whose histological pattern suggests both chondromyxoid fibroma and chondroblastoma
Cartilage-capped exostosis (osteochondroma), 512	1 23 45	1 : 1	Metaphyses of tubular bones and/or flat bones	Absent or pressure symptoms	Bony mass consisting of osseous tissue. Cortex of this lesion continuation of cortex parent bone. Bony mass surrounded by cartilage cap from which endochondral new bone forms, and from which a chondrosarcoma may originate	Arise from cortex, often pedunculated growing away from epiphysis. Tend to be sessile when flat bones affected. Growth usually ceases at puberty	Malignant change rare, more common with *multiple exostoses (diaphyseal aclasis)*

TABLE IV. *Classification of Bone Tumours and Tumour-like Lesions* (*contd.*)
(modified from the classification of the Royal National Orthopaedic Hospital, London, 1969)

IB. *Presumed to arise from skeletal connective tissue—forming* CARTILAGE (*contd.*)

Malignant

Tumour	Age of Incidence in Decades	Sex Incidence M F	Sites of Predilection	Clinical Features	Pathological Findings	Radiological Features	Remarks
Chondrosarcoma, 606	2 3 4 5 6 7	2 : 1	Innominate bones, femur, tibia and humerus, although thorax, spine, skull and maxilla may be affected. Lesions of long bones may be either diaphyseal or metaphyseal; metaphyseal predilection exists	Pain most frequent complaint, localised soft tissue mass common. Constitutional signs and symptoms usually absent in initial phase. Often history of long standing	Presumed to arise from peripheral or central cartilaginous foci with tendency for tumours of peripheral origin to appear deceptively benign in contrast to central lesions. Consider malignant if tissue is hypercellular, cell nuclei are plump, cells have multiple nuclei, nuclei are hyperchromatic and giant cartilage cells are present. Even with firm criteria, differentiation between benign and malignant cartilage tumours may be extremely difficult	Depend on anatomical location and origin—either primary or arising from cartilaginous precursor. Also peripheral or central *Peripheral* lesions originate from osteochondroma or parosteal chondroma; show evidence of enlargement with no clear-cut border or definition. *Central* lesions of appendicular skeleton show grossly destructive area with large, well-defined soft tissue mass. Endosteal new bone and endosteal scalloping common, particularly in tibia and femur. Varying degrees of calcification in approximately half the cases—occasionally amorphous but frequently punctate or circular. Extensive cortical thickening may be observed, due to organised periosteal reaction around long bones. Chondrosarcoma of flat bone tends to be grossly destructive, but frequently associated with varying amounts of reactive new bone	Large, well-defined soft tissue mass frequently observed—often larger in proportion to size of skeletal lesion than ordinarily anticipated. Soft tissue mass may be initial presenting radiological finding, particularly in pelvis. Skeletal metastases very rare but not unknown. Mesenchymal and juxtacortical chondrosarcomata represent special variants

TABLE IV. *Classification of Bone Tumours and Tumour-like Lesions (contd.)*
(modified from the classification of the Royal National Orthopaedic Hospital, London, 1969)

IC. *Presumed to arise from skeletal connective tissue—forming FIBROUS TISSUE*

	Tumour	Age of Incidence in Decades	Sex Incidence M F	Sites of Predilection	Clinical Features	Pathological Findings	Radiological Findings	Remarks
	Non-ossifying fibroma (fibrous cortical defect, metaphyseal fibrous defect), 508	**1** 2 3	2 : 3	Metaphyses of long bones, especially near knee	Usually absent, may fracture	Lesion consists of whorled bundles of spindle-shaped stromal connective tissue cells with varying amounts of interspersed intercellular collagenous material. Stromal cells may contain haemosiderin. Foam cells, containing lipid, and giant cells frequently present	Common. Eccentric translucent defects with narrow zone of transition and sclerotic margin. May thin and slightly expand cortex. Larger lesions may involve entire width of bone, e.g. fibula	Resolve by sclerosis. Biopsy rarely required. Carried by growth into diaphysis. Eventually replaced by normal bone.
	Juvenile fibromatosis, of infancy and childhood	1		Metaphyses of long bones. Occasionally flat bones	Two forms: benign and relatively aggressive, with soft tissue masses	Stromal connective tissue cells may suggest aggressive nature	Multiple, well-defined lucencies in metaphyses of long bones and in some flat bones	Soft tissue masses and pulmonary lesions worsen prognosis. Differs from rare entity of multiple non-ossifying fibromata
	Osteogenic fibroma	1		Tibia	Pain	Similar to fibrous tissue except for sheets of osteoid tissue	Resembles fibrous dysplasia, proximal half of tibia	Diagnosis essentially histological. ? aggressive form of fibrous dysplasia
Benign	**Parosteal (juxta-cortical) desmoid. 5**	1 2	2 : 1	Distal end of femur almost invariably, although similar lesion in other long bones rarely reported	May be asymptomatic. Localised pain	Fibroblastic proliferation and occasionally osteoid and osseous tissue. Hypercellularity may be present. Benign periosteal reaction. No real evidence of infective or tumorous tissue	Radiolucent defect and compact periosteal reaction posteromedial surface of distal end of femur. Localised soft tissue swelling rare and even more rarely punctate calcifications in adjacent soft tissue	Very likely not a true neoplasm, but secondary to trauma at musculotendinous insertion site of adductor magnus. Generally does not require biopsy for confirmation
	Desmoplastic fibroma, 1022	1 2 3 4	1 : 1	Long bones most commonly affected; innominate bone, scapula, clavicle, mandible and, rarely, a vertebra may be involved	Pain and local tenderness. Pathological fracture may be initial clinical manifestation. A rare tumour	Numerous, usually small fibroblasts with no mitotic figures or hyperchromatism. Fibroblasts generally embedded in collagenous, intracellular material with fibroblast-collagen ratio varying in different lesions. Nuclei small and elongated or large and plump. Histological pattern resembles soft tissue desmoids, juvenile aponeurotic fibroma, or even well-differentiated fibrosarcoma	Large, aggressive radiolucent lesion with endosteal erosion and cortical expansion. Pathological fracture not uncommon. Often wide zone of transition simulating fibrosarcoma. Irregular sclerotic resection around lesion occasionally. Trabeculated pattern not infrequent due to residual areas of cortical bone. Ends of long bones often involved	Radiological and histological distinction between desmoplastic fibroma and fibrosarcoma may be difficult. Difference in age groups important

TABLE IV. *Classification of Bone Tumours and Tumour-like Lesions* (*contd.*)
(modified from the classification of the Royal National Orthopaedic Hospital, London, 1969)

IC. *Presumed to arise from skeletal connective tissue—forming* FIBROUS TISSUE (*contd.*)

	Tumour	Age of Incidence in Decades	Sex Incidence M F	Sites of Predilection	Clinical Features	Pathological Findings	Radiological Features	Remarks
Benign	Calcifying juvenile aponeurotic fibroma, 1023	12		Palms of hands and soles of feet; occasionally on trunk	Localised pain and swelling	May resemble desmoplastic fibroma or low-grade fibrosarcoma	Stippled, calcific, soft tissue density involving palm of hand or sole of foot. Lesions may occur elsewhere (e.g. trunk)	Histological pattern may simulate desmoplastic fibroma and fibrosarcoma. Concept of 'pseudosarcoma' has been advanced
Malignant	Fibrosarcoma, 614	3456	1 : 1	Long bones or innominate bones commonest sites; approximately half the cases around knee, especially in proximal portion of tibia. Diametaphyseal predilection	Pain and swelling of some months duration	Pattern varies from poorly differentiated to well differentiated. May find spindle-shaped fibroblasts containing elongated nuclei in less malignant forms. Whorled and interlacing bundles of collagen fibres present. Undifferentiated lesions show excessive cellularity with anaplasia of fibroblasts—multiple nuclei and hyperchromatism. Necrosis, haemorrhage and secondary calcification may follow	Typically, highly destructive, expanding lesion, mainly medullary in location, with wide zone of transition and paucity of new bone formation. Infrequently, permeating pattern simulating round cell neoplasms. Periosteal reaction relatively slight and poorly organised. Codman triangles not infrequent. Well-defined soft tissue mass, although *smaller* than in Ewing's tumour and chondrosarcoma. Calcification occasionally secondary to necrosis and haemorrhage	May arise from thick, fibro-osseous wall of long-standing bone infarct. Highly anaplastic fibrosarcoma has poor prognosis; low-grade fibrosarcoma may resemble desmoplastic fibroma or giant cell tumour with distinctly better prognosis

ID. *Presumed to arise from skeletal connective tissue—forming* OSTEOCLASTIC TISSUE

	Tumour	Age of Incidence in Decades	Sex Incidence M F	Sites of Predilection	Clinical Features	Pathological Findings	Radiological Features	Remarks
Locally Malignant	Giant cell tumour, 564	34 56	5 : 6	Long bones most commonly affected, particularly distal end of femur, proximal end of tibia, distal end of radius, and proximal end of humerus. 60% around knee. Flat bones such as in-	Pain and swelling, often associated with trauma. Pathological fractures may occur. Age of patient of great importance. Very rare in immature skeleton	Consist of varying amounts and proportion connective tissue, stromal cells and giant cells. Stromal cells vary—plump, spindle-shaped or ovoid with large nucleus. Giant cells multinucleated with nuclei in centre. Proportion stromal cells to giant cells determines whether lesion benign or malignant. Tissue typing unreliable for prognosis	Osteolytic, eccentric lesion adjacent to articular surface of *adult* bone. Cortex thinned and expanded. Endosteal margin shows wide zone of transition. Lesion virtually always subarticular, even in flat bone	Exact cell of origin unknown, probably undifferentiated mesenchyme. Difficult to diagnose radiologically in unusual areas, e.g. patella, but basic criteria constant. Many benign tumours formerly regarded as

II. Tumours of Unknown Histogenesis

Name	No.	Sex ratio	Site	Clinical features	Pathology	Radiology	Remarks
(continued)			nominate bones and rib may be involved. Lesions in spine extremely rare, particularly confined to sacrum			Difficult to distinguish benign from malignant lesion radiologically. Approximately 10% of all giant cell tumours malignant. Lesions around wrist particularly suspicious	'variants', e.g. aneurysmal bone cyst, chondroblastoma. Pulmonary metastases have been reported from lesions histologically benign
Solitary bone cyst, 528	12	3 : 2	Proximal metaphysis of humerus (principally), femur, tibia, and less often flat bones such as calcaneus	Pain and swelling rare without pathological fracture. Often incidental finding	Cyst contains clear or yellowish serosanguineous fluid. Thin cortical wall usually present, composed of osseous tissue with often vascular connective tissue lining. Osteoid tissue and osseous trabeculae may be present, often with calcification and ossification and fibrin clots	Solitary, well defined, oval or round medullary translucency. Cortex thinned but only slightly expanded. Endosteal zone of transition narrow and sharply defined. May be multilocular. Carried by growth into diaphyses	'Fallen' fragment sign characteristic. Marked tendency to recur even after complete treatment by curettage and packing with bone chips, particularly in boys with large lesions. Cure anticipated when skeleton becomes mature. Reported incidence in innominate bones probably due to cystic degeneration in fibrous dysplasia
Epidermoid tumour of calvarium, 1072	234		Any bone of skull	Localised, painful swelling often, but may be asymptomatic	Squamous epithelium, keratin, cholesterol crystals characteristically present. Pathogenesis uncertain	Usually expanding, lytic, well-defined lesion with sclerotic border, which may be thick and dense. Mottled pattern with occasional areas of calcification or new bone. Soft tissue mass may be present. Tumour usually solitary, but satellite lesions may be observed	This lesion, often called 'pearly' tumour, must not be confused with cholesteatoma of petrous bone, which is associated with chronic mastoiditis. Epidermoid of skull may be congenital in origin
Ameloblastoma of jawbones, 578	245	3 : 2	80% in mandible, particularly affecting ramus and areas of the molar teeth; remainder in maxillae	Generally slowly-growing, locally-invasive lesion which may be discovered incidentally. Gradual, painless enlargement followed by ulceration and pain	Considerable variations exist in microscopic appearance. Two major types: *follicular* (more common)—columnar cells reminiscent of appearance of normal ameloblasts. Collagenised connective tissue may dominate picture. Microcysts observed. *Plexiform*—epithelial elements predominate with long cords of irregular masses of epithelial tissue bordered by columnar or cuboidal cells	Appearance varies greatly. Classical case shows multiple radiolucent areas varying in size and arranged in clusters radiating outward from central core. Less commonly, solitary lytic area without loculations. Occasionally, massive in size with reactive new bone, particularly in African natives	May show considerable growth potential, but malignant transformation and malignancy *ab initio* extremely rare

Benign

TABLE IV. *Classification of Bone Tumours and Tumour-like Lesions (contd.)*
(modified from the classification of the Royal National Orthopaedic Hospital, London, 1969)

II. *Tumours of Unknown Histogenesis (contd.)*

	Tumour	Age of Incidence in Decades	Sex Incidence M F	Sites of Predilection	Clinical Features	Pathological Findings	Radiological Features	Remarks
Benign	**Tumoural calcinosis, 872**	23	1 : 1	Adjacent to major joints—hip, knee, wrist, elbow, shoulder. Hands and feet infrequently	Familial tendency. Pain, swelling and disability. Firm, non-tender, freely movable mass generally palpated. Lesions may be solitary or multiple. No systemic effects	Mass cystic and multilocular, containing creamy white liquid resembling pus. Composed of calcium triple phosphate or carbonate suspended in albumin. Mononuclear or polynucleated giant cells rich in alkaline phosphatase often present histologically	Small, discrete, calcified nodules usually in soft tissues near or adjacent to joint initially. Nodules progress slowly later to well-defined, lobulated, calcified masses. Osseous involvement rare except in region of elbow where erosion distal end of humerus may occur	Entity must be distinguished from bursal calcification, post-traumatic soft tissue mineralisation and metastatic calcification observed with various endocrine abnormalities (particularly after renal transplants) and collagen disorders. Calcifying neoplasms of soft tissue also to be differentiated
Locally Malignant	**Adamantinoma of long bones, 572**	45 6	1 : 1	Mid-shaft of tibia; other long bones very rarely	Mild pain of long duration, possibly localised swelling. Pathological fracture may occur	Epithelial and endothelial origins suggested—latter more likely. Cellular structure varies. Polygonal or spindle-shaped cells with alveolar or tubular arrangement. Also may show less cellular pattern with considerable collagenisation, suggesting sarcoma. Squamous transformation of tumour cells with definite epithelial pearls simulating squamous cell carcinoma also occurs. Lesion usually highly vascular	Generally eccentric, expanding, lytic area typically thinning cortex of middle third of tibia. Lesion may be multilocular with wide zone of transition and poor definition of endosteal margins. Reactive new bone may be present. Satellite translucencies characteristic. Tibia and fibula may be affected simultaneously	Lesion is locally malignant and tends to recur after surgical treatment. No relationship to ameloblastoma of mandible. Cortical fibrous dysplasia and adamantinoma may coexist in same tibial shaft, but frequently lesion represents true adamantinoma with elements suggesting fibrous dysplasia
Malignant	**Ewing's tumour, 619**	12 3	5 : 4	Entire skeleton, but mainly long bones, spine and innominate bones	Localised pain, pathological fracture, anaemia, weight loss and other signs and symptoms related to generally fatal disorder	Varied histological pattern. Usually fields of tumour cells of uniform appearance in vacuolated cytoplasmic material. Cells poorly delineated, containing round nuclei. Small polyhedral cells with clear-cut borders containing small, dark nuclei (pyknosis) with pale cytoplasm indicate degenera-	*Long bones.* Mottled, permeating, destructive pattern involving medulla with wide zone of transition. Adjacent cortex frequently permeated and destroyed. Lesion tends to be	Skeletal and pulmonary metastases frequently and early. May be confused with other round cell lesions—metastases from neuroblastoma, primary reticulum cell sarcoma,

tion. Cells frequently perithelial around vessels ('rosette formation'). Necrosis, haemorrhage and new vessel formation may occur. New bone (non-malignant) may form

elongated, with diaphyseal predilection in at least three-quarters of cases. Classical concentric 'onion-skin' periosteal layering considered specific for Ewing's tumour encountered relatively infrequently. Large, sharply-defined soft tissue mass as in chondrosarcoma, frequent finding *Flat bones*. Permeating destructive pattern also particularly innominate bone. New bone formation common. In spine, vertebral body may show destructive, mottled appearance and gross collapse

metastases from carcinoma, myeloma. Age of patient important

IIIA. *Presumed to arise from other skeletal components*—BLOOD AND LYMPH VESSELS

			Sites	Clinical	Macroscopic/Microscopic	Radiology	Comments
Benign	**Aneurysmal bone cyst, 532**	*123*	1 : 1	Spine, innominate bones particularly common. Major long bones often affected. Even tubular bones of hands and feet, calcaneus, clavicle and skull (rarely)	Acute, severe, progressive, localised pain, probably attributable to infraction. Spinal lesions may produce neurological defects and even paraplegia	Grossly bulging shell of bone with periosteal reaction containing large, distended, thin-walled, blood-filled, cystic cavities, almost invariably without blood clots. Histologically, muscular coats absent in blood vessel walls, lined by endothelial cells and multinucleated giant cells, haemosiderin and phagocytes.	Eccentric, expanding, osteolytic lesion destroying overlying cortex of which a remnant only may remain as shell. Zone of transition usually narrow with reactive sclerosis, but may be wide, suggesting aggressive nature	Important to differentiate from giant cell tumour and osteoblastoma, especially in spine Arteriogram may show hypervascular pattern around periphery of neoplasm, but no true tumour vessels Aetiology debatable. Trauma suggested by some. Underlying lesions may coexist and be responsible for development of aneurysmal bone cyst

TABLE IV. *Classification of Bone Tumours and Tumour-like Lesions* (*contd.*)
(modified from the classification of the Royal National Orthopaedic Hospital, London, 1969)

IIIA. *Presumed to arise from other skeletal components*—BLOOD AND LYMPH VESSELS (*contd.*)

Tumour	Age of Incidence in Decades	Sex Incidence M F	Sites of Predilection	Clinical Features	Pathological Findings	Radiological Features	Remarks
Haemangioma, 518	2 3 45 6	1 : 2	Three sites: (1) spine (most common); (2) skull; (3) long bones and other flat bones	Depend on site but often incidentally detected. Pain or swelling may be present. Pathological fracture occasionally, particularly vertebral body	*Spine:* Thin-walled, dilated vascular channels set in substratum of fatty marrow which may be gelatinous. No definite connective tissue capsule. Many osseous trabeculae resorbed; remainder thickened, running vertically. Lining of vascular spaces—single layer endothelial cells. *Skull:* Thin-walled, blood-filled, vascular spaces starting in diploe. Trabeculae may be coarse or honeycombed. New bone between vascular spaces giving 'spoke-wheel' pattern. *Long bones and other flat bones:* Variable. Tends to resemble lesions in skull. Two types generally described—cavernous and capillary	*Spine:* Coarse vertical striations in vertebral bodies and occasionally appendages without enlargement. May cause compression fracture and even extradural block on myelography. *Skull:* Osteolytic areas with 'sunburst' appearance, with narrow zone of transition. Large, adjacent vascular channel common. *In other flat bones or long bones:* Characteristic 'sunburst' or reticulated appearance, resembling calvarial lesions. Residual bone trabeculae within lesion tend to be thick and dense	Lesions tend to be expansile *except* in vertebral bodies. Wide spectrum of vascular tumours of skeleton exists. Multiple lesions occur and even widespread skeletal involvement (cystic angiomatosis and 'vanishing bone' syndrome of Gorham) must be considered part of pattern of skeletal haemangiomata
Cystic angiomatosis of bone, 1113	2 3	2 : 1	Multiple bones involved including skull, ribs, innominate bones, spine and femora. Distribution predominantly axial; peripheral lesions relatively uncommon	Often diagnosed as incidental finding, although pain at skeletal site may be present with or without pathological fracture. Soft tissue angiomata may produce localised masses and swelling	Endothelial-lined spaces may be vascular, lymphatic or both. Difficult to determine tissue of origin histologically. Multilocular cystic lesions vary from 1 to 2 mm to several cm in diameter and are lined by endothelium and intercommunicate. Telangiectasia may be observed at periphery of bone lesions. ?Vascular hamartomata	Multiple, well-defined, round or oval lytic lesions with thin sclerotic borders. Predominantly axial skeleton. Periosteal reaction rare. Vertebral lesions show no vertical striations as in vertebral haemangiomata. Soft tissue angiomata may be present with phleboliths. Other sites of involvement include spleen, lungs, liver, pericardium, and	Rib best bone for biopsy. Lymphography may be abnormal in areas of soft tissue involvement. Arteriography generally of no value. Prognosis usually poor when spleen involved. Otherwise bone lesions rarely cause serious complications

Benign

	Tumour	No.	Ratio	Site	Clinical features	Pathology	Radiology	Comments
							retroperitoneal space. Anterior mediastinal masses of haemangiomatous or lymphangiomatous origin and chylous pleural effusion may be observed	
Benign	**Massive osteolysis ('vanishing bone' syndrome of Gorham), 1110**	34	1 : 1	Major long bones, innominate bones, thorax and spine, although no bone immune to involvement. Short tubular bones of hands and feet also affected	Autosomal dominant inheritance suspected but not documented. Patient often presents with dull aching and weakness in limb. Pathological fracture and consequent deformity may be prominent features. Involvement of spine and thorax may lead to death from neurological and pulmonary complications. History of trauma often elicited, but significance doubtful	Bones soft and spongy with irregular eroded cortical margins. Fibroblastic reaction uncommon. Defective bone replaced by loose angiomatous tissue consisting of capillary or sinusoidal vessels. Lymphangiomatous elements may predominate. Marrow spaces of bone show hypervascularity of a reactive type. Osteoclastic activity depends on stage of process	Depend on stage of disorder. Initially subcortical and intramedullary radiolucent foci followed by expanding intramedullary lytic areas without sclerosis. Fractures commonly precede stage of massive bone resorption, resulting in tapering margins of ends of bone fragments with typical cone-shaped configuration. No evidence of bone repair	Angiographic studies generally not helpful, although increase in blood flow suggested. Pointed bone ends after pathological fracture may suggest pseudarthrosis of neurofibromatosis or fibrous dysplasia. Therapy generally unsuccessful, although spontaneous remission reported
Locally malignant	**Haemangiopericytoma, 1115**	3456		Spine, pelvis, major long bones	Pain and swelling	Related to glomus tumour which may be variant. Arterial walls in tissue abnormally thin and lined with polyhedral (epithelioid) cells which are probably smooth muscle in origin and have been called the pericytes of Zimmerman. If abundant, tend to call lesion haemangiopericytoma, if sparse, glomus tumour	Usually bone-destroying. No characteristic pattern. Difficult to distinguish benign from malignant lesion	Cannot be diagnosed radiologically except by exclusion. High malignant potential
Benign or malignant	**Glomus tumour, 1115**	3456	1 : 2	Rare in bones. Terminal phalanges of fingers especially affected	Stabbing pain of long duration. Hypersensitivity to thermal changes	See above. Typically, electron microscopy shows epithelioid smooth muscle cells and mast cells	Rare. Clear-cut area of destruction, usually small, related to soft tissue mass	Differentiate from implantation dermoid cyst
Malignant	**Angiosarcoma (haemangioendothelioma), 1870**	125		Long bones, especially femur and tibia	Pain and swelling	Typical lesion contains anastomosing vascular spaces lined by atypical round or ovoid endothelial cells. Reticulin surrounding cords can be demonstrated by special silver stains. If highly anaplastic may resemble fibrosarcoma	Rare. Purely destructive, rapidly growing, 'soap bubble' expansion. Lung metastases early. Never arises from a haemangioma	Regarded by some as simply a highly vascular osteosarcoma

TABLE IV. *Classification of Bone Tumours and Tumour-like Lesions (contd.)*
(modified from the classification of the Royal National Orthopaedic Hospital, London, 1969)

IIIB. *Presumed to arise from other skeletal components*—NERVE TISSUE

	Tumour	Age of Incidence in Decades	Sex Incidence M F	Sites of Predilection	Clinical Features	Pathological Findings	Radiological Features	Remarks
Benign	**Solitary neurofibroma, 63** (For neurofibromatosis see Table IB)		1 : 1	Cervical and dorsal spine; auditory canal	Nerve pressure symptoms. Soft tissue masses	Appear in subcutaneous tissue, along peripheral nerves and at or near medullary junctions. Various sub-groups include Schwannoma (nuerinoma, neurilemmoma)—arise from sheath cells. Whorled nodule consisting of linear patterns. Schwann cell nuclei mucinous or connective tissue matrix. Fibrillar whorls with radiating nuclei formed in palisades	Pressure erosion of adjacent bone. Usually only of importance in bony canals, especially exit foramina of spine, which are enlarged. Soft tissue mass produces 'dumb-bell' tumour. 8th nerve may be affected	Arises from non-specific nerve sheath. Tumours of the specific nerve sheath (neurilemmoma) cause identical radiological changes. Intra-osseous neurofibroma rarely encountered in major long bone, spine, mandible. Characterised by presence of localised pain and point tenderness. Well-defined, lucent lesion in medullary cavity, radiologically
Malignant	**Neurogenic sarcoma, 59**	345		None	Pain and massive swelling	Commonly represents malignant degeneration in a neurofibromatous lesion. Considered fibrosarcoma by some pathologists, but others believe such lesions of Schwannian origin. Highly cellular and fasciculated lesions. General types: (1) sclerosing (2) spindle cell (3) anaplastic	Infiltrating destructive process. Wide zone of transition. Large soft tissue mass	10% of patients with generalised neurofibromatosis develop malignant neurogenic tumour

IIIc. *Presumed to arise from other skeletal components*—NOTOCHORD

	Tumour	Age of Incidence in Decades	Sex Incidence M F	Sites of Predilection	Clinical Features	Pathological Findings	Radiological Features	Remarks
Locally Malignant	**Chordoma, 638**	3456	3 : 2	Sacrum—55%; skull—25%; spine—20%, especially C2	Localised pain, neurological deficits, soft tissue mass with lesions of spine. Intracranial signs and symptoms referable to chordomata of clivus	Varied appearance. In *immature* type tissue may be highly cellular with no vacuolation in cytoplasm of cells. Cells in such tissue small, round and well outlined. In *mature* type distended cells containing vacuoles (physaliphorous cells), enmeshed in considerable	Central osteolytic destruction. Zone of transition usually narrow. Large associated soft tissue mass with flecks of calcification. May be very extensive and provoke	Derived from vestigial notochord In lesions of spine, myelography may show extradural defects and even complete block Metastases rare but may occur in later

			mucin. Lesion may on occasion suggest undifferentiated fibrosarcoma or chondrosarcoma. Calcification and even ossification may occur	bizarre new bone formation Lesions of clivus may simulate pituitary adenoma, meningioma or metastasis	stages, although skeletal metastases exceptional

IV. Tumours of Synovial Tissue

Benign	**Synovial chondromatosis, 870**	345	2 : 1	Knee most commonly. Hip, ankle, wrist, shoulder and other major joints affected	Low grade, chronic pain, swelling, limitation of motion, limp and 'locking'. Localised tenderness may be present	Cartilage masses demonstrated grossly in subserous layer of synovial membrane. These may calcify or even ossify. Cells microscopically arranged in small clusters. Nuclei generally normal but may be hyperchromatic, plump and irregular	Small, stippled, faintly calcified (initially), nodules generally no larger than several millimetres in diameter and usually of similar size, in and around affected joint with evidence of synovial thickening and/or effusion. Nodules may ossify in later stages. Secondary erosion of intracapsular bone, including articular surfaces, not uncommon. Joint space narrowing and osteophyte formation may occur in late stages.	Often confused with post-traumatic joint degeneration with calcified and ossified loose bodies, which tend to be larger than opacities in synovial chondromatosis and vary more in size. Probably true neoplasm. Differentiate from pigmented villonodular synovitis, in which calcification virtually never occurs
	Pigmented villonodular synovitis, 558	34	3 : 2	Knee most commonly affected. Other joints involved include hip, ankle, wrist, shoulder and joints of hand and foot	Mildly painful, chronic swelling of affected joint area	Aetiology unknown. Synovium of affected joint shows reddish or yellowish-brown nodular clumps with appearance suggesting 'scraggly beard'. Microscopically, pigmented synovial lining cells in nodules bordering clefts. Cells may contain haemosiderin pigment granules and lipid. Nucleated giant cells, fibrosis and collagenisation common. Similar findings in tenosynovial and bursal lesions	Synovial thickening with large erosions of capsular attachments. Endosteal margins tend to have narrow zones of transition. Serial studies show very slow progression. Large 'lakes' corresponding to erosions shown on arthrography Well-defined erosions with sclerotic borders on both sides of a joint characteristic	Formerly regarded as benign synovioma or xanthomatous giant-cell tumour, but tumourous nature of lesion not firmly established. May also involve bursae and tendon sheaths. Calcification in lesion virtually unknown Characteristic subarticular erosions more common in tightly compartmentalised joints—e.g. hip, hallux

TABLE IV. *Classification of Bone Tumours and Tumour-like Lesions* (*contd.*)
(modified from the classification of the Royal National Orthopaedic Hospital, London, 1969)

IV. *Tumours of Synovial Tissue* (*contd.*)

	Tumour	Age of Incidence in Decades	Sex Incidence M F	Sites of Predilection	Clinical Features	Pathological Findings	Radiological Features	Remarks
Malignant	**Synovioma (synovial sarcoma), 640**	3 4 5 6	2 : 3	Any major joint, especially knee. Also joints of foot	Pain and swelling	Characteristically 2 types of cells in varying proportions. (1) synovial type, plump or elongated cells in sheets or cords lining clefts or slits (2) sarcomatous stromal cells (primitive cells) resembling fibrosarcoma, spindle cells contained within reticulin or fibrin. Cells lining clefts may be cuboidal or columnar, suggesting epithelial tumour. If sarcomatous stromal cells predominate, correct diagnosis may be missed. Clefts contain mucoid material. Necrosis and calcification may occur	Destructive lesions usually on both sides of joint with irregular margins and much soft tissue thickening. Amorphous calcification not uncommon	May also affect tendon sheaths, again often with diffuse calcification

V. *Tumours of fatty tissue origin*

	Tumour	Age of Incidence in Decades	Sex Incidence M F	Sites of Predilection	Clinical Features	Pathological Findings	Radiological Features	Remarks
Benign	**Lipoma (soft tissues), 1030**	3 4 5 6 7	1 : 1	Usually in subcutaneous tissues—most often back of neck, axilla and upper limbs. May be solitary or multiple	Localised mass, mild pain. May be asymptomatic	Typical fat cells, although variation of cellular pattern may exist from adult plump cells to small polyhedral variety. Considerable amount of fibrous tissue may be present in lesion. Mass usually surrounded by thin, fibrous capsule with interspersed fibrous strands coursing through fatty tumour. Lesion often highly vascular	Appearance will depend on relative amount of fibrous tissue within lesion. If tumour mainly consists of fat, will be lucent; if fibrous tissue is present in abundance, may have lesser degree of lucency; or none at all. Calcification relatively uncommon. Erosion of adjacent bone rare. Periosteal reaction infrequent	Synovial lipoma called 'lipoma arborescens'. *Macrodystrophia lipomatosa*, although characterised by deposition of fatty masses in soft tissues, belongs with group of phakomatoses Lipoma may occur in spinal canal
	Parosteal lipoma, 1030			Generally affects long bone—femur, tibia or humerus	Usually slowly enlarging soft tissue mass. May be asymptomatic unless pressure on adjacent nerve	Consists of lobulated fatty mass with fibrous tissue present between lobules and with cartilage and bony proliferation. Tumour adherent to shaft of adjacent bone, arising from periosteal layer	Lobulated, translucent areas of fat separated by curvilinear strands of bony density observed adjacent to long bone shaft. Periosteal proliferation usually evident	May be considered analogous to parosteal chondroma, although a much less common lesion

				Clinical	Pathology	Radiology	Comments
Benign	**Intra-osseous lipoma, 1030**			Long bones most commonly affected—metaphyseal predilection	Lesion often discovered incidentally	Lesion typically a mass of mature adipose tissue within medullary cavity of affected bone. Interspersed bony trabeculae frequent. Metaphyseal predilection. Infarction of surrounding bone not common	Well-defined lytic lesion with residual trabeculae resulting in loculated pattern. Bone sclerosis uncommon and periosteal reaction generally absent, unless pathological fractures supervene. Cortical expansion common. Calcifications within lesion may be present	Intra-osseous lipoma very rare (Jaffe has denied existence). Suggestion has been made that lesion is derived from infarct of bone. Potential for malignant transformation extremely rare
	Liposarcoma of soft tissues, 1031	567	2 : 1	Thigh, popliteal fossa, leg, gluteal region, retroperitoneal tissues. Tendency for deeper soft tissues to be affected	Painful soft tissue mass, usually slowly growing	Nodular mass, often encapsulated, containing tumour tissue with variable appearance. Mixture of mature fat cells and myxoid tissue containing lipoblasts, which may be spheroid, spindle-shaped or 'signet ring' in appearance. Highly anaplastic lesions may show few mature fat cells and often lipoblasts and myxoid areas with many mitotic figures. Rounded vacuolated cells may be present. May resemble fibrosarcoma	Usually relatively opaque lesion in contrast to benign lipoma because of more solid tissue component. Ossification and calcification often present, comparable to parosteal lipoma. Calcification in relatively dense soft tissue mass should arouse suspicion of this neoplasm. Pressure erosion of adjacent bone common feature. More aggressive lesions may enlarge rapidly; these often do not cause pressure erosion of bone nor do they show calcification and ossification	In past a less aggressive type of liposarcoma was described as fibromyxoma
Malignant	**Intra-osseous liposarcoma, 1032**			Humerus, ulna, fibula, tibia and innominate bones	Not distinctive—pain and local swelling common	Very large, fat-containing tumour cells with solitary and multiple bizarre nuclei. Cells usually contain foamy cytoplasm. Myxomatous or fibrosarcomatous pattern may be present. Lesion may vary from highly anaplastic form with many mitotic figures to well differentiated appearance. On occasion may resemble renal cell carcinoma	Lesion predominantly grossly destructive, although low-grade tumours may be well defined. Generally no gross calcification radiologically	As in instance of benign counterpart (intra-osseous lipoma) Jaffe has doubted authenticity of this neoplasm

TABLE IV. *Classification of Bone Tumours and Tumour-like Lesions* (*contd.*)
(modified from the classification of the Royal National Orthopaedic Hospital, London, 1969)

VI. *Skeletal Metastases presented in order of frequency of primary tumour* (*see text for detail.* **586**)

Tumour	Age of Incidence in Decades	Sex Incidence M F	Sites of Predilection	Clinical Features	Pathological Findings	Radiological Features	Remarks
Breast	4 5 6 7	+	Predominantly axial skeleton	Often asymptomatic. Vague pain. Pathological fracture	Trabecular resorption predominant by malignant cells of primary tumour. Non-malignant new bone may be formed. Generally applies to all types of metastases listed below	70% *osteolytic*. Multiple and large but diffuse osteolytic infiltration resembling osteoporosis may occur. *Mixed* 20%. *Osteoblastic* 10%. Lytic lesions may sclerose after oophorectomy and male hormone therapy	To be considered with any porotic spinal collapse in elderly females, possibly with spinal cord compression. Rarely expanding lesions in pelvis, mixed osteoblastic and osteolytic type
Lung (Bronchus)	5 6 7	4 : 1	Entire skeleton, including hands and feet	Pain, pathological fracture. Occasionally asymptomatic	Occasionally expansile. Rarely, blastic, particularly with carcinoid, **1088**	Mainly *osteolytic* with no sclerotic reaction. Initially may have narrow zone of transition. Often solitary	Chest film advisable with any suspected skeletal neoplasm over age 40. Also with hypertrophic osteoarthropathy. May invade ribs directly (Pancoast tumour). Some purely blastic and mixed lesions
Prostate	5 6 7 8	+	Axial skeleton especially pelvis and spine. Some appendicular lesions, especially bizarre in tibia	Often an incidental finding. Vague pain. Acid phosphatase elevated	Predominantly osteoblastic. Occasionally mixed. Lytic in older age group. May cause 'ivory vertebra'	Mainly *osteoblastic*. Multiple oval or round areas of density enlarging and merging. Exceptionally, solitary destructive lesions or sun-ray spiculation. Arrest or regression with female hormone therapy	Solitary vertebral lesions may simulate Paget's disease but do not produce the characteristic enlargement of that disease. Lytic areas in elderly
Kidney (renal cell carcinoma)	5 6 7	3 : 2	Axial skeleton common. Spine, pelvis, ribs may be affected. Also major long bones	Localised pain. Pathological fracture common	See above. Lesions tend to be focal and few in number. Widespread dissemination rare	Frequently solitary *osteolytic* lesion, characteristically *expanding* and provoking relatively little new bone formation. Wide zone of transition. Spread is rarely diffuse	Likely to simulate primary malignant neoplasms, especially giant-cell tumour if subarticular. Vascular pattern on arteriography accentuated

Very commonly Metastasising to Skeleton

Very commonly Metastasising to Skeleton	**Sympathetic nervous system. (Neuroblastoma)**	1 2		Whole skeleton	Young children.	Catecholamines in urine. Joint pain may simulate arthritis. Constitutional symptoms severe	Extensive diffuse destruction especially in metaphyses. Skull sutures widened by marginal tumour infiltration. Usually little reactive sclerosis, but exceptionally solitary lesions develop 'sun-ray' spiculation or extreme density	Closely resembles changes of leukaemia, **784**
	Ewing's tumour, 619	**12** 3	5 : 4	Whole skeleton	Severe illness. Pain, loss of weight, fever, anaemia. Pathological fracture	See under primary tumour	Multiple lesions, each comparable to primary tumour	Rapidly fatal
	Colon	5 6 7	3 : 2	Haemopoietic portions of skeleton	Pain and tenderness at site of involvement	See above. Mainly destructive; reactive new bone not uncommon	Predominantly lytic lesions with wide zones of transition. Occasionally bone forming, simulating metastases from carcinoma of prostate	Lesions in left side of colon (and rectum) more apt to metastasise to skeleton
Commonly Metastasising to Skeleton	**Thyroid**	**56** 7		Axial skeleton, femur, humerus	Pain, pathological fracture, local pulsation, on account of hypervascularity	See above	Predominantly osteolytic with wide zone of transition. Expanding lesions common, simulating plasmacytoma	May appear many years after thyroidectomy. Tumours often of very low-grade malignancy with slow growth of metastases. May resemble metastases from renal cell cancer—highly vascular on angiography

TABLE IV. *Classification of Bone Tumours and Tumour-like Lesions (contd.)*
(modified from the classification of the Royal National Orthopaedic Hospital, London, 1969)

VI. *Skeletal Metastases presented in approximate order of frequency*

Tumour	Age of Incidence in Decades	Sex Incidence M F	Sites of Predilection	Clinical Features	Pathological Findings	Radiological Features	Remarks
Commonly Metastasising to Skeleton							
Bronchial carcinoid	4 **5 6 7**	2 : 3	Predominantly axial skeleton	*Carcinoid syndrome*—flushing, cyanosis, rash, diarrhoea, abdominal pain, enlargement of liver, asthma, fluctuations in blood pressure, tendency to peptic ulceration and increased incidence of pulmonary stenosis and tricuspid insufficiency. Hepatic metastases usually present when carcinoid syndrome encountered Gastrointestinal carcinoids very rarely metastasise to skeleton. Approximately 10% of bronchial carcinoids metastasise	Key substance in pathogenesis of carcinoid syndrome is serotonin 5-hydroxy tryptamine. Increased levels of 5-hydroxy indoleacetic acid detected in urine Bronchial carcinoids histologically identical to gastrointestinal carcinoids, but less likely to contain argentaffin granules. Bone sclerosis represents secondary response to carcinoid cells in marrow cavity	Generally diffuse, sclerotic process involving skeleton. Lesions usually slowly progressive	Cases occasionally encountered in which osteoblastic skeletal metastases remain unchanged for many years with patient in apparently good health. Metastases frequently observed from carcinoids histologically benign
Infrequently Metastasising to Skeleton							
Rectum	**5 6 7**	2 : 1	Haemopoietic portions of skeleton	Localised pain. Pathological fractures may occur	See above. Mainly destructive; infrequently, reactive new bone	Most often lytic lesions with wide zone of transition	May be asymptomatic. Blastic lesions may simulate closely a primary osteosarcoma. Age of patient important
Stomach	**5 6 7**	2 : 1	Haemopoietic portions of skeleton	Localised pain; may be asymptomatic	See above. Often reactive new bone associated with destructive lesions	Bone forming or mixed lesions not uncommon, although purely lytic metastases may be observed	Surprisingly high incidence of purely blastic lesions

Primary site		Sex ratio	Part of skeleton affected	Symptoms	Reactive bone	Lytic / blastic character	Remarks
Urinary bladder	567	3 : 2	Entire skeleton	May be asymptomatic	See above. Mainly destructive but reactive new bone not uncommon	Often *lytic* when confined to bladder; *blastic* when prostate involved	More frequently present than suspected. Not uncommonly responsible for bizarre lesions in tibia and fibula, simulating fulminating infective lesions or primary malignant neoplasms
Uterus (corpus, cervix)	4 567	+	Haemopoietic portions or skeleton	Pain and tenderness, although lesions may be asymptomatic	See above. Mainly destructive; reactive new bone infrequently	Generally lytic, with occasional mixed or sclerotic pattern, particularly with lesions from cervix	Expanding lesions may simulate metastases from kidney. Metastatic lesions in innominate bones not uncommon. Destructive adjacent lesions in more than one bone of pelvis should suggest direct spread—not uncommon
Testis	34		Haemopoietic portions of skeleton	Often painful, particularly backache with spinal lesions. May be asymptomatic	See above. Mainly destructive, but reactive new bone often	Predominantly lytic, but occasionally bone forming lesions may occur, simulating metastases from carcinoma of the prostate	Blastic lesions from seminoma not uncommon
Melanoma (predominantly of skin)	4 567	2 : 1	Entire skeleton	May be asymptomatic, but generally painful	See above	Generally lytic and often expanding, simulating metastasis from renal cell carcinoma	More frequently present than suspected
Nasopharynx (Schmincke tumour)	345		Haemopoietic portions of skeleton	May be asymptomatic but usually localised bone pain	See above. Mainly destructive, occasionally reactive new bone	Lesions may be lytic or bone-forming, with surprisingly high incidence of sclerotic lesions	Direct invasion of sphenoid sinuses and sella turcica not uncommon
Ovary	567	+	Predominantly axial skeleton	Localised pain, but often asymptomatic	See above	Mainly destructive lesions. Blastic metastases rare	A neoplasm recognised with increasing frequency
Vascular neoplasms Haemangiosarcoma (includes malignant haemangiopericytoma) from various sites			Haemopoietic portion of skeleton	Localised pain	See above. Mainly destructive	Generally lytic, often expanding lesions	Wide spectrum of vascular neoplasms exists (see text)

Infrequently Metastasising to Skeleton

Rarely Metastasising to Skeleton

The metastases which occur *rarely* from a variety of primary foci are listed in the text on page 586. It should be appreciated that unusual primary tumours tend to produce unusual metastases

TABLE V. *Metabolic and Endocrine Disorders*

Disease	Clinical Features	Common Sites	Pathological Features	Radiological Features	Remarks
Osteoporosis, 700	Senile and post-menopausal types most common. Also occurs with scurvy, Cushing's syndrome and thyrotoxicosis (q.v.). Idiopathic form in young adults	Axial skeleton especially. Immobilisation of limbs	Diminished osteoid formation associated with (1) inadequate supply of protein, vitamin C; (2) hormonal imbalance (sex hormone deficiency, adrenocortical or thyroid excess); (3) reduced activity	Diffuse decrease in bone density. Involutional change in elderly. Diagnosis frequently depends on exclusion of other entities. Vertebral body collapse common	Sudeck's atrophy (post-traumatic painful osteoporosis). Paralytic states engender osteoporosis
Scurvy, 670	Maternal vitamin C protects for first six months. Occurs then in infants and young children. Rare in adults. Pain and swelling ends of long bones, spontaneous bleeding various sites (teeth etc.), pallor and anaemia. Diminution vitamin C concentration in blood plasma and in urine after load test	Early evidence in knees and ankles but ends of other long bones involved. also anterior ends of ribs	Inadequate supply vitamin C (ascorbic acid). Diminished production and maintainence of intercellular ground substance. Osteoid formation reduced—trabeculae thin (osteoporosis)—capillary walls weakened. Metaphyses exceedingly fragile with uneven, widened chondro-osseous junction with condensation of calcareous material. Metaphyseal injuries may separate epiphyses and cause extensive capillary bleeding into muscles, joints and subperiosteal areas of diaphyses	Following series of radiological changes: (1) generalised osteoporosis; (2) impaired osteoid formation with continued deposition calcium phosphate in osteoid formed—produces 'white' line adjacent to epiphyseal plate; (3) rings of increased density around relatively lucent epiphyses; (4) zone of attrition metaphysis (Trümmerfeld zone); (5) metaphyseal fractures, especially in weight-bearing long bones, with 'corner' sign; (6) haematoma elevates periosteum with subsequent calcification and ossification which may be concurrent	Must be differentiated from 'traumatised' child. In adults, only osteoporosis with vertebral compression observed
Cushing's syndrome (hypercorticism), 707	Weakness, hypertension, impotence or amenorrhoea, diabetes, obesity, water retention causing oedema, virilism with facial hirsutism and acne and psychiatric episodes. Diminution of appreciation of pain, fractures common, often relatively or completely asymptomatic. Joint instability may resemble neuropathy. Bone infections may also be asymptomatic	Generally axial skeleton. Spine, ribs and major joints particularly involved. Appendicular skeleton not exempt. Skull late	Associated with excess production of cortisone and hydrocortisone, increase in pituitary corticotropin and hyperplasia or neoplasia of adrenal cortex. May also be iatrogenic. Effects on multiple systems (not considered here). Skeleton shows varying degrees of osteoporosis due to diminution osteoblastic function. Secondary necrosis of bone and degenerative joint disease due to overt or subclinical trauma. Bone condensation at fracture sites—particularly vertebrae and ribs—prominent feature. Bioassays show increase corticotropic activity. High blood sugar and chloride, low P and alkalosis	Diffuse osteoporosis with peculiar mottling of skull. Relatively painless infractions and gross fractures common with considerable 'pseudocallus'. Biconcave vertebral bodies. Joint derangement may be comparable to true neuropathy. Bone and joint infections may be relatively asymptomatic without significant sclerotic response	While Cushing's syndrome of natural origin is relatively rare, iatrogenic effects of steroid therapy are not uncommon, with relatively asymptomatic fractures, neuropathies and bone and joint infection. Similar joint lesions often associated with other analgesics

Hypophosphatasia, 1082	Represents heritable disorder (autosomal recessive) of bone metabolism of varying severity. Defective skeletal mineralisation resembling rickets with low serum and tissue levels of alkaline phosphatase and urinary excretion of phospho-ethanolamine which is substrate for alkaline phosphatase. Clinical severity and prognosis vary. *Neonatal form*—many infants stillborn or die within six months. Irritability, convulsions, vomiting, respiratory distress, fever and failure to thrive common. Infants small with short, bowed extremities, large joints and soft cranial bones. *Infantile form*—similar clinical signs between second week and sixth month of life. Most in this group survive. Hypercalcaemia and signs of impaired renal function common, due to renal interstitial fibrosis. *Childhood form*—presents between six months and two years of age. Bowed legs, knock-knees, late onset of walking, skeletal pain, premature loss of teeth and severe dental caries characteristic. *Adult form*—actual fractures may be presenting complaint in adults. Clinical signs and symptoms minor. Familial history often obtained	Virtually entire skeleton, but most important radiological features in long bones and skull	Excess amino acid, phosphoethenolamine, in urine. Changes typical of osteomalacia on bone biopsy	Varies with type but in neonatal and infantile forms particularly. Profound defective mineralisation with large irregular metaphyseal defects mainly around wrists, knees and costochondral junctions. Skeleton at birth severely affected. Newborn skeleton may be almost completely unossified. Fractures common. Cranial sutures widened with premature craniosynostosis. Metaphyses of long bones show findings typical of rickets. Osteoid seams common in adults.	Infantile and early childhood forms may be differentiated from other forms of rickets as well as metaphyseal dysostosis by specific laboratory findings Minor radiological changes may be observed in asymptomatic or mildly affected siblings. Represents an important cause of refractory rickets. More common than appreciated
Familial hyperphosphatasemia, 1056	Usually in children and young adults. Autosomal recessive inheritance suggested. Siblings may be affected. Striking predilection for Puerto Ricans. Usually progressive enlargement of the skull initially followed by bowing of limb bones. May develop hypertension because of increased vascularity of bone. Death possible by encroachment of hyperostotic masses on trachea and pharyngo-esophagus	Virtually entire skeleton may be affected—mainly haematopoietic portion	Laboratory studies demonstrate sustained elevation of alkaline and acid phosphatase of blood serum, elevation of blood uric acid and aminopeptidase. Laboratory data indicate increased turnover of skeletal collagen. Confirmed by tetracycline labelled radionuclides studies Disorder characterised by failure of primitive fibrous tissue to mature into compact Haversian bone. Widened cortex with thin, primitive trabeculae	Increase in size of long bones with severe modelling deformities. Cortical surfaces of long bones thickened and sclerotic. Medullary cavities and spongiosa tend to be wide and coarse in appearance. Cyst-like lesions in metaphyses. Pseudo-fractures or actual fractures not uncommon with bowing deformities of long bones. Skull thickened in membranous portion with spheroid areas of bone sclerosis. Base of skull (preformed from cartilage) and facial bones essentially normal	Young individuals diagnosed as Paget's disease probably examples of this entity Thyrocalcitonin may be effective therapeutically

s

TABLE V. *Metabolic and Endocrine Disorders (contd.)*

Disease	Clinical Features	Common Sites	Pathological Features	Radiological Features	Remarks
Hyperostosis corticalis generalisata (Van Buchem's disease), 1060	Rare, hereditary, systemic disorder autosomal recessive in type, described in both children and adults with no sexual predilection. Appearance of patients suggests acromegaly with particularly prominent clavicles and mandible. Facial paralysis, hearing and visual disturbance common due to bony encroachment on foramina of skull	Skull, mandible, clavicle, ribs, innominate bone, long bones and tubular bones of hands and feet characteristically affected. Spine usually spared	Increased serum alkaline phosphatase generally. Other laboratory data unrewarding. In one case mature lamellar and cortical new bone demonstrated. Bone marrow normal. Studies with polarised light non-contributory	Diffuse sclerotic process affecting cortex and medulla of involved skeletal segments, obliterating clear demarcation between these areas. Bony excrescences may be evident on shafts of long bones	Relationship of this disorder to familial hyperphosphatasemia has been suggested, but not established. Of great importance is the presence of primitive woven bone histologically in hyperphosphatasemia as opposed to mature bone noted in Van Buchem's disease, suggesting that the two disorders are different
Osteomalacia, 652	Common factors—irritability, bone pain, tenderness, deformities, e.g. bow legs, rachitic rosary. Major causes include (1) deficiency states; (2) gastroenterogenous disorders; (3) organic renal disease; (4) tubular dysfunction states; (5) hypophosphatasia; and (6) miscellaneous (see text)	In *growing* skeleton—metaphyses of long bones, particularly around wrists, knees and ankles. Also skull and spine if due to renal disease. In *adult* skeleton—pelvis, ribs, scapulae, thoracic spine, major long bones and short tubular bones less often	Osteomalacia characterised by inadequate osteoid mineralisation. (Contrast *osteoporosis*—failure to form osteoid tissue.) Osteomalacia in growing skeleton known as *rickets*. Causes of failure to mineralise osteoid tissue: (1) calcium deficiency; (2) inadequate vitamin D—dietary deficiency or failure to absorb or use; (3) excessive phosphate excretion; (4) diminished absorption of fats, normal vehicle for fat-soluble vitamin D; (5) bile salt deficiency required to emulsify fat prior to absorption; (6) deficiency of alkaline phosphatase. Laboratory findings vary with cause. Major disease groups: (1) dietary rickets in infants; (2) adult dietary form (famine osteomalacia); (3) vitamin D resistant rickets (possibly due to renal tubular dysfunction states); (4) gastroenterogenous (steatorrhoea); (5) renal osteodystrophy (glomerular type I); (6) renal osteodystrophy (glomerular type II); (7) hypophosphatasia	*Growing skeleton (rickets):* wide zones of translucency and irregularity of epiphyseal plates. Weight-bearing areas show splaying and bowing of metaphyses. Skeleton shows reduced density. Periosteal reaction may occur. 'Bossing' of calvarium in severe cases. Epiphyseal centres poorly mineralised and may be absent. Osteoid seams (Looser's zones) relatively uncommon in children. *Adult osteomalacia. Looser's zones* pathognomonic—residua of stress fractures which may be asymptomatic. Tend to be symmetrical, affecting chiefly obturator rings of pelvis, lower ribs, inferior borders of scapulae, major long bones (often femoral necks) and metatarsals. Generalised diminution bone density with marked softening producing bowing of long bones, spinal deformities and basilar invagination of skull. Late effects osteomalacia in spine may result in paraspinal ligamentous calcification and ossification, reminiscent of ankylosing spondylitis	Many of the radiological changes of osteomalacia are attributable to secondary hyperparathyroidism

Primary hyperparathyroidism (HPR), 676	Usually in middle-aged with slight predilection for women. Rare instances observed at birth. May be asymptomatic. Four general groups: (1) discovered incidentally as part of routine examination; (2) clinical effects related to urinary tract—nephrocalcinosis; (3) effects of hypercalcaemia (constipation, muscular weakness, etc.); (4) skeletal lesions (pain and pathological fracture). Extensive structural deformities now rare. May be part of a pluriglandular disorder (Werner's syndrome)	Hands, outer ends of clavicle, long bones (upper femora and tibiae), ischial tuberosities, pubis. 'Brown' tumours common ribs, pelvis, long bones, tubular bones of hands	Laboratory studies helpful—hypercalcaemia, hypophosphataemia, hypercalciuria and hypophosphaturia—although need not be abnormal. Excessive production parathyroid hormone. Benign (usually chief cell) adenoma of one parathyroid gland usually responsible, although multiple glands may be involved. Skeletal effects: bone destruction due to increased osteoclastic activity, absorption of trabeculae and subsequent cyst ('brown tumour') formation, fibrosis, haemorrhage, necrosis and numerous giant cells	Approximately 20% of patients show skeletal lesions. Now diagnosed much earlier. Hand commonest site—subperiosteal resorption middle phalanges 2nd and 3rd fingers, also outer ends of clavicle, medial surfaces femoral necks and tibiae, ischial tuberosities, pubic bones, sacroiliac joints and dorsum sellae. 'Brown tumours' may be markedly expanding, simulating neoplasms. Pathological fractures through 'brown tumour' may be the initial manifestation which may stimulate localised skeletal changes. Subperiosteal resorption of phalanges almost invariably evident if any other skeletal lesions identified	Increased bone density rarely—may be associated with anabolic effects of parathormone. Angiography useful in establishing location and size of hypervascular parathyroid adenoma. Radioimmunoassay techniques of venous blood may provide definitive diagnosis. Congenital form exists. Certain neoplasms may produce parathormone-like substance (e.g. lung)
Secondary hyperparathyroidism (HPR), 682	Age and clinical presentation depend on cause. Organic renal disease and renal tubular dysfunction states commonly responsible. Skeletal pain may occur. Rachitic-like deformities common in children. Associated with changes of osteomalacia in children and adults	Similar to primary hyperparathyroidism	Diminished excretion of phosphate occurs with consequent elevation of blood serum phosphorus. Serum calcium at or near normal limits. Serum alkaline phosphatase usually elevated. Diminished vitamin D content probably necessary for skeletal expression of both primary and secondary hyperparathyroidism. Excessive parathormone production needed for compensatory purposes. Generally due to hyperplasia parathyroid glands. Stimulus probably due to increased serum phosphorus or decreased serum calcium. Histological findings similar to primary form. 'Brown tumours' relatively uncommon in contrast to primary HPR, but occur. Metastatic soft tissue and arterial calcification usually extensive	Subperiosteal resorption as in primary form. 'Brown tumours' relatively unusual. In childhood, epiphyseal plates widened and distorted and metaphyses disorganised (renal rickets). Associated osteoporosis. Severe generalised demineralisation and bowing of limb bones common. 'Ruggerjersey' effect in spine due to associated new bone formation. Calvaria thickened. Metastatic calcification soft tissues and arteries common in terminal stages. Calcific deposits also in subcutaneous tissues, periarticular areas, lungs, heart and liver. Tumoural calcinosis simulated. Meniscal calcifications in joints, e.g. knee, infrequent in contrast to primary HPR	New bone formation may be prominent feature, producing generalised increase in bone density. May be difficult to separate radiological features of osteomalacia and secondary HPR in same patient. Renal osteodystrophy is combination of osteomalacia, secondary HPR and osteoporosis
Hypoparathyroidism, 1189	Generally short stature, dry coarse skin, loss of hair, atrophy of nails, round facies and cataracts. Tetany characteristic. Mental retardation on occasion if chronic. Females more commonly affected	Entire skeleton may be affected although changes usually minimal	Results from inadequate amounts of parathormone, either from lack of adequate secretion or from loss or removal of parathyroid. Also observed in infants of mothers with compensatory hyperparathyroidism. In idiopathic form parathyroid gland replaced by fat. Results in absence or decrease of parathormone with response of hypocalcaemia to administration of this hormone	Minimal skeletal changes. Increased density or osteoporosis generally difficult to demonstrate. Calvarial thickening, premature fusion of ossification centres and paraspinal ligamentous calcifications occasionally. Abnormal dentition frequent, consisting of delay in development or eruption, hypoplasia, thickening of lamina dura. Basal ganglia calcification more common than in PH	Basal ganglia calcification may be secondary to degenerative process or an incidental finding. Need not reflect hormonal abnormality

TABLE V. *Metabolic and Endocrine Disorders* (*contd.*)

Disease	Clinical Features	Common Sites	Pathological Features	Radiological Features	Remarks
Pseudohypopara-thyroidism (PH), 1188	Short stature, thick-set individuals, obesity, round face, mental retardation, cataracts, hypocalcaemic tetany refractory to parathormone	Hands, skull, calvarium, soft tissues of extremities and occasionally long bones and spine	Excessive secretion of parathormone by often hyperplastic parathyroid glands. Serum hypocalcaemia and hyperphosphataemia with no response to parathormone administration	Most common characteristic skeletal abnormalities in hands and feet, with shortening of metacarpals, metatarsals and phalanges, which is usually disproportionate in hands. 'Cone' epiphyses and premature fusion may occur. Exostoses encountered in diaphyses of long or short tubular bones. Thickened calvarium, soft tissue calcification and occification in half the patients, mainly in skin, subcutaneous tissues, facial planes, ligaments and tendons. Periarticular areas commonly affected. Calcification basal ganglia and dentate nuclei of cerebellum in third to half of patients. Dentition abnormal in half of patients	Increased endogenous production of parathormone with absence of normal end-organ response primarily in the kidney but to some extent also in bone
Pseudopseudo-hypoparathyroidism (PPH), 1188	Small stature, obesity, round face, mental retardation less frequent than in PH and occasionally tetany	Appendicular skeleton (hands and feet) and calvarium	Blood chemistries normal	Short metacarpals and metatarsals. Calvarial thickening occasionally. Soft tissue calcification relatively infrequent in contrast with PH. Basal ganglia calcification uncommon. Dentition normal	Both PH and PPH probably represent different clinical expressions of same genetic disorder
Hypothyroidism (cretinism), 690	Mild to severe forms. Classically in advanced cases—gross mental and physical growth retardation. Characteristic facies, thick skin, protruding tongue. Mild forms may show only slight dwarfing. Specific and rapid response to treatment with thyroid. Radio-isotope scanning procedures with I-131 diagnostic	All bones of extremities, spine and skull principally. Entire skeleton may be affected	Congenital cretinism or acquired juvenile myxoedema results from diminution or absence thyroid secretion. May be due to thyroid dysgenesis or absence or hypoplasia of thyroid. Goitrous cretinism due to iodine deficiency. Genetic basis possible, creating metabolic error. In endemic cretinism may find nodular goitre with areas microscopically of compensatory hyperplastic changes	Dwarfism, delayed skeletal maturation (Greulich and Pyle), multicentric major ossification centres, particularly femur and humerus, abnormalities of spine—tongue-shaped vertebral bodies, generally entire spine with kyphos thoracolumbar area. Skull changes—persistent sutures, Wormian bones and delayed development base, nasal bones and teeth	May be confused with dysplasia epiphysealis multiplex, bilateral Perthes' and several of the mucopolysaccharidoses
Acromegaly, 718	Before puberty—*gigantism*. After skeletal maturation—*acromegaly*. Typical acromegalic—increase in stature (if young), coarse features, thick skin, enlargement hands and feet, protruding jaw, 'barrel' chest,	Skull, spine, hands, feet, thorax	Due to excess production of growth hormone, usually because of eosinophilic adenoma or occasionally simple hyperplasia of anterior lobe of pituitary. Enlargement of all organs produced. Osseous overgrowths of osteochondral junc-	Reflect excessive skeletal growth. *Skull.* Enlarged sella turcica and paranasal sinuses, hyperostosis, prognathism. *Spine and thorax.* Large vertebral bodies with peripheral accretion new bone and posterior 'scalloping', enlargement	Early radiological signs of importance: sesamoid index (thumb), 'heelpad' sign and posterior concavities lumbar vertebral bodies. *Gigantism* causes generalised skeletal overgrowth

	Clinical features	Skeleton affected	Pathology	Radiology	Differentiation
	headaches and visual disturbances. Increase pituitary growth hormone on assay studies		tions, vertebral bodies and articular bone ends hands and feet. Hyperplasia of connective tissues occurs	anterior ends of ribs. *Appendicular skeleton*. Soft tissue thickening and tufting terminal phalanges, enlargement of sesamoids; increase of joint spaces by cartilage hypertrophy	without distinctive features
Hypopituitarism, 727	Pituitary dwarfism results from impaired function of anterior lobe pituitary, of unknown cause. Lack of end-organ response. *Simmonds syndrome* is term applied to hypopituitary state in adults; mainly in women. Human growth hormone (HGH) deficiency produces growth failure with onset in infancy or early childhood. Growth may not be complete until 4th or 5th decade. Secondary sex characteristics under-developed. Round, doll-like facies with normal sized head. Height generally more retarded than weight. Hypoglycaemia present and plasma HGH levels low	Entire skeleton, including skull	Growth of cartilage and bone arrested. Epiphyseal cartilage persists; compact layer of bone formed in metaphyses. Epiphyses remain unfused into adult life	Delay in skeletal maturation, with unfused ossification centres into middle adult years. Evidence of tumour destruction around pituitary fossa may be present if neoplasm is cause	Must be differentiated from other forms of dwarfism associated with dysplasias and dystrophies
Effects of Poisoning. 732 **Fluorosis, 740**	Generally asymptomatic until middle adult life except for discolouration, hyperplasia, and premature decay of teeth. Stiffness of joints may simulate ankylosing spondylitis. Secondary anaemia may occur. Evaluation of urinary fluorine content helpful. Haematological studies generally normal Chronic fluoride intoxication occurs in geographical areas where fluorine content of drinking water exceeds 4 to 8 parts per million. Other causes relate to workers in various industries	Principally haematopoietic skeleton—mainly innominate bones and lumbar spine. Long bones infrequently affected. Skull rarely, if ever, involved	Pathological changes in skeleton consist of absence of nuclei in osteocyte lacunae, suggesting impaired viability. Bone resorption demonstrated. Apposition of new bone by osteoblasts accounts for characteristic osteosclerosis, only apparent after long periods of exposure—25 to 30 years	Earliest characteristic changes in innominate bones and lumbar spine, with coarsening and thickening of trabecular pattern, followed by homogeneous increase in bone density. Roughening of muscle attachments, particularly ischial spines and iliac crests, with calcification of pelvic ligaments. When long bones affected periosteal reaction and bony excrescences may occur. Osteosclerosis of appendicular skeleton observed only rarely	Unusual and interesting cause of florid periosteal reactions described as effect of chronic fluoride poisoning in wine drinkers (fluorides have been used as preservatives for wines) Differential diagnosis includes myeloid metaplasia and diffuse osteoblastic metastases
Lead, 733	Types: (1) *Alimentary*: vomiting, intestinal colic (2) *Neuromuscular*: weakness and paralysis (3) *Encephalopathic*: restlessness, lethargy, signs of raised intracranial pressure. Lead lines in gums. Mental retardation serious hazard	Metaphyses of growing skeleton	Lead *ingested* by eating lead paint (tastes sweet) or drinking water contaminated by lead pipes. *Inhaled* by dust or fumes (e.g. burning old battery cases). Deposited in metaphyses, impregnating trabeculae composed of considerable cartilage with acidophilic giant cells. Calcium to some extent replaced but reactive bone also forms	Bands of increased metaphyseal density in children. Almost unique in proximal end of fibula and inferior angle scapula. Intermittent episodes may resemble growth lines. Cortex and flat bones may be slightly dense. Modelling deformities later, e.g. flask-shaped femur. Widened skull sutures. ?lead in G.I. tract	Condition not rare, especially in Southern United States. Encephalopathy and mental retardation particularly important, possibly without radiological evidence. No radiological changes observed in adults

TABLE V. *Metabolic and Endocrine Disorders (contd.)*

Disease	Clinical Features	Common Sites	Pathological Features	Radiological Features	Remarks
Bismuth, Phosphorus, Arsenic, 733	Features similar to lead	Growing metaphyses	*Bismuth* from anti-syphilitic medication in past. May be transmitted to foetus	Similar dense metaphyses and intermittent transverse densities in long bones, diaphyses and iliac wings	Rarely encountered
Radium, 736	Bone pain, anaemia, secondary malignancy in later years	Haemopoietic skeleton	Radium salts formerly used as medication (1910-1930). Areas of bone necrosis from β radiation and repair	Lytic areas due to necrosis and fibrosis. Scattered and poorly defined. Secondary new bone formation as repair process. Sarcomatous metaplasia as complication later in life	Localised bone necrosis of maxilla and mandible formerly an occupational hazard in luminous dial painters using radium compounds
Cadmium, 732	Effects of renal disease and osteomalacia	Whole skeleton	Cadmium ingested in contaminated water or inhaled in production of electric batteries. Renal damage	Typical changes of osteomalacia resulting from nephropathy	Only recently recognised as industrial hazard
Occupational acro-osteolysis (Vinyl Chloride), 1026	Symptoms reminiscent of Raynaud's phenomenon with scleroderma-like skin changes hands (and even feet). Clubbing of fingers may be present	Principally hands, but feet may be involved similarly. Occasionally sacro-iliac joints may also be affected and infrequently other skeletal areas	No definitive data. In one case reported changes in defective skin with disruption and fragmentation of collagen and elastic fibres. Intimal fibrosis and hypertrophy of small vessels reported. No histological studies of affected bone	In typical case acro-osteolysis of terminal tufts of one or more fingers. Earliest change loss of cortex of tuft of distal phalanx followed by small half-moon cut in cortex of tuft—slice effect'. In more advanced stages extensive destruction with complete loss of tuft. Fibrous or bony repair in healing phase. Erosive and sclerotic changes both sacroiliac joints reminiscent of ankylosing spondylitis. Lytic lesions may occur elsewhere in skeleton	Entity occurs in individuals employed in manufacture of vinyl chloride polymers, particularly those who perform cleaning of reactors by hand. Haemangiosarcoma of liver reported recently in individuals exposed to vinyl chloride (not observed in association with skeletal lesions)
Vitamin A intoxication, 1164	Two forms: *Acute*: Vomiting and other signs of increased intracranial pressure. skeletal pain and alopecia. Bulging of fontanelles. *Chronic*: Does not occur before one year of age. Failure to thrive with loss of appetite, pruritus and fretfulness. Tender, hard swellings on extremities, jaundice, hepatomegaly, splenomegaly, alopecia and dry skin. Haemorrhagic manifestations	*Acute*: Skull. *Chronic*: Long bones of extremities and tubular bones particularly of feet. Diaphyses characteristically involved. Skull also affected	In experimental animals excess of vitamin A accelerates maturation and degeneration of epiphyseal cartilage. Osteoclastic activity increased with multiple fractures	*Acute*: Reminiscent of pseudo-tumour cerebri with widening of cranial sutures. No other skeletal changes. *Chronic*: Cortical thickening of long bones and tubular bones mainly affecting diaphyses. Evidence of increased intracranial pressure	Permanent stigmata may occur—short stature, disparity in growth of paired limb bones and flexion deformities of lower extremities. Splaying and cupping of metaphyses and irregularity of margins of ossification centres together with premature fusion may result
Vitamin D intoxication, 1165	Two forms: *Acute*: Occurs because of ingestion of enormous amounts of vitamin D. Symptoms and signs referrable to central nervous system, dehydration, fever.	Periarticular soft tissues and long bones	Normocytic, normochromic anaemia. Elevated blood serum calcium and phosphorous and alkaline phosphatase. Deposition of calcium in periarticular soft tissues, blood vessels, tubules of kidney and oc-	Metastatic calcification in virtually any soft tissue structures, but particularly periarticular areas. Increased depth of provisional zone of calcification of growing skeleton, with generalised osteoporosis and thicken-	May have relationship to supravalvular aortic stenosis associated with idiopathic hypercalcaemia of infancy due to abnormal sensitivity of infant to vitamin D

Disease	Symptoms	Sites	Pathology	Radiological changes	Remarks
(continued)	Pain at multiple skeletal sites. *Chronic:* A number of organ systems affected: gastrointestinal (diarrhoea, etc.); central nervous system (vertigo, headache, convulsions and even coma); psychiatric (depression, etc); urological (frequency, nocturia, etc.); and ophthalmological (impairment of vision)	casionally other organs. Cystic lesions in periarticular areas		ing of cortical surfaces of long bones. Alternating bands of increased and diminished density of long bones in later stages. Falx cerebri frequently calcified	
Ochronosis (alkaptonuria), 1046	Observed first 3 decades of life. Grey, brown or yellow pigmentation sclerae, cornea and skin with bluish discolouration cartilaginous structures—nose and ear. Symptoms caused by degenerative joint changes—mainly shoulders and hips in relatively young patients with 2 : 1 predilection for males over females. Initial symptoms generally spinal. Progressive stiffening of spine common although pain generally less severe than in ankylosing spondylitis	Intervertebral discs, spine, shoulders, hips	In absence of homogentisic oxygenase—homogentisic acid accumulates in various body tissues, being excreted in urine and sweat. When deposited in tissues oxidises to form brownish-black granules which are deposited in deeper layers of articular cartilage, with synovial thickening and cartilaginous metaplasia resulting. Subchondral sclerosis, cysts, eburnation and osteophyte formation around joints characteristic. Chondrocalcinosis infrequent. In spine, narrowing and calcification of intervertebral discs with marginal osteophytes. Secondary calcification in ear, nose, bursae, tendon sheaths, and other areas	May precede onset of symptoms. Reflect pathological changes. Extensive degenerative joint disease shoulders and hips and degenerative disc disease in spine in young patients. Calcifications in bursae and tendon sheaths and ear and nasal cartilages. Intervertebral disc calcification with thinning of disc spaces common and most diagnostic feature. Associated osteoporosis frequent. Meniscal calcifications and calcified loose bodies in major joints with degenerative joint disease	Diffuse intervertebral disc calcification and premature degenerative joint disease should suggest this unusual, and sometimes familial entity
Gout Chondrocalcinosis (pseudogout)	These essentially metabolic disorders are summarised on page 2026 (Table VII)				
Wilson's Disease (hepatolenticular degeneration), 1048	Rare disorder inherited as autosomal recessive whose basic abnormality is congenital disturbance of copper metabolism. Usually recognised during first three or four decades of life. Renal tubules affected with osteomalacia. High concentrations of amino acids, protein, glucose and phosphates in urine Neurological symptoms, including tremor, etc., initially. Pathognomonic ring of brown pigment around limbus of cornea (Kayser-Fleischer ring). Degenerative joint disease at unusually early age	Wrist, metacarpophalangeal joints, hips and knees most commonly affected, although associated osteomalacia may produce widespread skeletal abnormalities	Excess of copper deposition lenticular region of brain and liver which may cause cirrhosis Decrease of serum ceruloplasmin causes increase of copper concentration in many tissues	Associated osteomalacia produces generalised demineralisation and frank radiological evidence of osteomalacia with Looser's zones or rickets depending on the age of patient. Irregularity of articular surfaces of joints ('fringing') and later subchondral fragmentation commonly observed. Chondrocalcinosis also occurs.	Analogy has been made with haemochromatosis which is due to excessive iron deposition. Excessive copper probably affects cartilage and subchondral bone. Severe premature degenerative changes in affected joints observed in later years

TABLE V. *Metabolic and Endocrine Disorders* (*contd.*)

Disease	Clinical Features	Common Sites	Pathological Features	Radiological Features	Remarks
Homocystinuria, 1102	Considerable variation in severity of abnormalities. Lenticular dislocation, mild to moderate mental retardation, cavus deformities of feet and valgus deformities of knees, tendency to thrombosis of arteries and veins. Malar flush, high arched palate, dental abnormalities, sternal deformities and aortic arch abnormalities	Entire skeleton may be affected	Represents connective tissue abnormality. Defect in structure of collagen or elastin representing inborn error of methionine metabolism, due to deficiency of cystathionine synthetase, resulting in excessive accumulation of homocystine	Scoliosis common with marked curvatures. Osteoporosis widespread particularly in spine, producing biconcave vertebral bodies and concave cavities of posterior surfaces of vertebral bodies. Involvement of metaphyses with mild coxa valga and humerus varus. Widening of distal end of ulna with enlargement of capitate and hamate bones and punctate calcified and ossified deposits in epiphyseal plates of wrist frequent. Dilatation of aortic arch and dissection of aorta may be present; pectus carinatum and excavatum may be observed in chest film.	Many cases diagnosed as Marfan's syndrome are actually homocystinuria. Tendency to thrombosis in arteries and veins constitutes serious threat to life
Marfan's syndrome, 1102 (More probably congenital, but often confused with homocystinuria)	Many *forme fruste* examples. Dislocation of ocular lens, aneurysm of aorta and overgrowth of long bones most conspicuous features. Spinal scoliosis, muscular hypoplasia and hypotonicity, contractures of fingers. Varying deformities of feet, visceral hernia, cardiovascular and mitral valve abnormalities	Appendicular skeleton	No known chemical abnormality. Probably represents connective tissue abnormality due to defect in structural collagen or elastin, producing collagen which is more soluble and mechanically inadequate	Include elongation of long bones and tubular bones of hands and feet; disproportionately elongated extremities in relationship to trunk. Thin, cortical margins of long bones. Severe scoliosis with widening of neural canal. Pectus excavatum deformities, large aortic arch and possible evidence of dissecting aneurysm and other types of heart disease	Arachnodactyly, although commonly associated, need not be present in Marfan's syndrome. Must not be confused with homocystinuria

TABLE VI. *Diseases of the Haemopoietic System and Marrow* (including Reticuloendothelial Storage Disorders)

A. DISEASES PRIMARILY INVOLVING RED BLOOD CELLS

Pathological Condition	Age in Decades	Sites of Predilection	Clinical Features	Pathological Findings	Radiological Features	Remarks
Thalassaemia (Mediterranean or Cooley's anaemia), 746	1 2 3	Red marrow areas (i.e. whole skeleton in child, regressing with survival to axial skeleton). Compensatory extramedullary haemopoiesis with hepatosplenomegaly	Chronic anaemia, dyspnoea, pallor, fatigue, jaundice from destruction of abnormally fragile red blood cells. Rodent facies, cardiac enlargement and terminal failure. Sexual development retarded	Due to abnormalities haemoglobin molecule. Anaemia severe, small RBC, many nucleated. Also polychromasia, basophilic stippling, increase in reticulocytes, Howell-Jolly bodies. Foetal Hb present-HbF, deficiency-HbA. Bone marrow becomes profoundly hyperplastic in haemopoietic and also appendicular skeleton. Thickening of calvarium with hyperplasia of maxilla. Extramedullary haemopoiesis very common in posterior mediastinum	*Marrow hyperplasia:* Coarse medullary texture, many trabeculae destroyed, overlying cortex thinned and expanded. Hence biconcave metacarpals, flask-shaped femora, other errors of trabecular modelling. *Skull* at first shows widened diploic space, then thickening of outer table, rarely with hair-brush' spiculation. Hyperplasia impedes sinus development, causing rodent or mongoloid facies, malocclusion of teeth. Cardiac enlargement. With survival, peripheral areas revert to normal or are slightly dense	Wide geographical distribution from Mediterranean eastwards. Hereditary incidence in persons having such racial origin. Abnormal haemoglobin molecule. *Major* form with homozygous trait (both parents). *Minor* with heterozygous (one parent)—changes mainly less severe and survival more common
Thalassaemia variants Haemoglobin/sickle cell disease, 746	1 2 3 4 5 6 7 8	Red marrow areas, but radiological changes likely to be central in skull and spine	Same features but much less prominent or even absent in mild forms	Comparable to above in lesser degree	Survival in a state of balance common. Peripheral bones normal. Spine likely to be porotic. Skull affected in same way but less prominently	Crossing with other abnormal haemoglobins and sickle cell trait not uncommon
Sickle cell anaemia, 750	1 2 3 4 5	All bones initially affected but often not enough to cause x-ray change. Infarcts in long bones mainly. Also salmonella infection. Later reactive sclerosis peripherally and skull thickening	Features of chronic anaemia with frequent skeletal and abdominal crises due to *infarction*. Can also cause mongoloid facies. Essentially confined to black race	Several varieties. Sickling trait may be crossed with normal or abnormal haemoglobins (usually with A or C) or even thalassaemia. Heterozygous forms less severe than homozygous. Erythrocytes when deprived of oxygen become long and slender. Anaemia and jaundice result. Altered red cells result in stasis, anoxia, thrombosis and infarction many organs. Bone infarcts common, particularly spine, femoral and humeral heads, hands and feet. Erythropoietic hyperplasia initially causes widening spongiosa, cortical thinning. Changes not as marked as in thalassaemia. Extramedullary haemopoiesis less common. Subendosteal new bone common in late stages	In black *infants* below age of 2 periosteal reactions on small bones of hands and feet suspicious. In children minor infarcts cause areas of density and even lesions like Perthes' disease. Massive infarction simulates acute osteomyelitis, but without the clinical features, with fairly rapid repair. Sometimes associated with salmonella infection. *Adults* show bone infarcts, especially in humeral and femoral heads, diffuse trabecular thickening and endosteal new bone apposition. Spinal osteoporosis with partial vertebral cupping very important sign	Endosteal bone apposition may give appearance of 'bone within a bone'. Spinal changes due to bone infarcts. Lesions in hands (and feet) formerly considered salmonella infection mainly due to infarction

TABLE VI. *Diseases of the Haemopoietic System and Marrow (contd.)*
(including Reticuloendothelial Storage Disorders)

A. DISEASES PRIMARILY INVOLVING RED BLOOD CELLS *(contd.)*

Pathological Condition	Age in Decades	Sites of Predilection	Clinical Features	Pathological Findings	Radiological Features	Remarks
Erythroblastosis foetalis, 1144	At birth	Long bones	Excessive foetal haemolysis results in haemolytic jaundice, anaemia, petechiae, ecchymosis, mucosal bleeding and hepato-splenomegaly	Rh positive foetal erythrocytes may cause isoimmunisation of Rh-negative pregnant women. Foetal haemolysis caused before birth, producing jaundice and anaemia. Cells formed mainly erythroblastic, but may observe myelocytes and mega-karyocytes. Oedema, serous effusions, liver damage and extramedullary haemopoiesis main effects. Marrow hyperplasia with severe anaemia. Kernicterus of central nervous system, especially basal ganglia	Translucent metaphyseal bands affecting long bones with adjacent bands of increased density. Suggests disturbance in endochondral formation of bone in foetus. Transient 'ghost' lines in vertebrae may be present Foetal hydrops most severe form of erythroblastosis foetalis, characterised by marked generalised oedema of soft parts with pleural, pericardial and peritoneal effusions. Obliteration of foetal fat line of foetus radiologically due to marked subcutaneous oedema, side-to-side displacement of foetus *in utero* and deformity of foetal thorax. Peculiar posture of limbs because of oedema	Replacement transfusion techniques remarkably successful in treatment, stressing importance of diagnosis by radiologist *in utero* Abnormal antigen-antibody reaction between mother and foetus causes massive haemolysis
Iron deficiency anaemia and other abnormalities of erythroblastic tissues. 'Bahima' disease, 747	1	Skull	Anaemia caused by inadequate diet	Invariably infants and children. Due to inadequate diet, impaired G.I. absorption, excessive bleeding. New bone requires considerable iron (stored at birth). If anaemia of new-born (physiological) persists due to inadequate supply iron, marrow hyperplasia occurs. Mainly evident diploë calvarium—red marrow sites	Skull only involved. No reports of more extensive changes. Facial bones normal without distortion of antra by marrow hyperplasia	Similar changes have been noted with cyanotic congenital heart disease and with polycythaemia vera. Latter condition occasionally responsible for bone infarcts especially in femoral head, 1147

B. DISEASES PRIMARILY INVOLVING WHITE BLOOD CELLS

Pathological Condition	Age in Decades	Sites of Predilection	Clinical Features	Pathological Findings	Radiological Features	Remarks
Leukaemia *Childhood*, **784**	**1 2**	Axial skeleton, major long bones. Bone changes in 50%	Invariably acute. Fever, malaise, bone pain. May simulate rheumatic fever, rheumatoid arthritis	Virtually always acute. Stem cells not always identifiable. Marrow spaces packed with leukaemic cells which destroy trabeculae in spongiosa and infiltrate cortex, rarely causing trabecular thickening. Atrophy of trabeculae due to pressure leukaemic cells causes osteoporosis. Metaphyseal bands caused by depression endochondral function and later destruction by leukaemic cells. Periosteal reaction result of stimulation periosteal osteoblasts by leukaemic cells	Horizontal lucent bands metaphyses, periosteal reaction, osteoporosis; cortical and medullary erosions and occasional intense reactive new bone formation	Metastatic neuroblastoma may present similar radiological pattern
Leukaemia *Adults*, **785**	**2 3 4 5 6 7**	May be myelogenous, lymphocytic or monocytic. Haemopoietic skeleton, mainly spine pelvis and major long bones	Usually chronic. Weakness, splenomegaly, anaemia. Abnormal W.B.C. count with immature forms	Several varieties. Commonest, *myelogenous* and *lymphatic*. Skeletal manifestations radiologically in chronic forms—lymphatic more frequent. Osseous resorption due to leukaemic cells commonest manifestation. Osteolysis—destruction trabeculae in spongiosa—may occur. Leukaemic cells beneath periosteum produce periosteal reaction. Marrow fibrosis and new bone formation may occur long-standing cases	Skeletal findings relatively infrequent. Mainly osteoporosis, radiolucent mottling cortex and spongiosa, compression fractures vertebral bodies	Skeletal changes in acute leukemia of adults recently observed relatively often. Similar spectrum of radiological abnormalities as in childhood form except for rarity of metaphyseal lucent bands.
Myeloid metaplasia (myelosclerosis, myelofibrosis), 790	**4 5 6 7 8**	Whole skeleton. Liver and spleen usually, but not invariably enlarged	Initially myelofibrosis with chronic anaemia from reduction of haemopoietic tissue	Replacement of marrow by fibrous connective tissue initially with thickening of bone trabeculae later. Results in marked variations blood cellular elements—leukaemic-like picture, marked normocytic, normochromic anaemia with immature forms red and white cell series. Extramedullary haemopoiesis most marked in spleen, but may occur in posterior mediastinum and other sites	Marrow fibrosis initially causes radiolucent pattern. Diffuse increase of density due to sclerosis of fibrous tissue thickening trabeculae. Marrow spaces narrowed by endosteal new bone apposition. Patchy translucencies due to partial persistence of fibrous tissue. Control films necessary in early stages	Probably a leukaemic variant, although relatively benign, but terminal leukaemia common. May follow polycythaemia vera, especially after P32 therapy. Radiotherapy to be avoided

TABLE VI. *Diseases of the Haemopoietic System and Marrow (contd.)*
(including Reticuloendothelial Storage Disorders)

B. DISEASES PRIMARILY INVOLVING WHITE BLOOD CELLS (contd.)

Pathological Condition	Age in Decades	Sites of Predilection	Clinical Features	Pathological Findings	Radiological Features	Remarks
Mastocytosis (mast cell disease), 1038	23	Mainly haemopoietic skeleton	Benign and malignant forms exist, divided into cutaneous mastocytosis and systemic mastocytosis. Urticaria pigmentosa characteristic (10% of such patients show skeletal lesions in contrast to 70% of patients with systemic mastocytosis) Symptoms and signs of carcinoid syndrome common—flushing, headache, tachycardia, hepatosplenomegaly, lymphadenopathy, anaemia, leukopenia, leukocytosis, and thrombocytopenia not infrequent. Haemorrhagic tendencies may exist	Related to the effect of proliferating mast cells which are of mesenchymal origin and infiltrate the skin producing pigmented rash of urticaria pigmentosa. Cells elaborate heparin, histamine, serotonin and hyalo-uronic acid, suggesting unicellular endocrine gland. In skeleton excess of mast cells produces fibroblasts and granulomatous foci which replace bone marrow and trabeculae resulting in osteoporosis, followed by generalised osteosclerosis	Vary greatly. Circumscribed and diffuse forms of skeletal lesions exist *Circumscribed*—lytic or blastic lesions often in long bones, innominate bones and skull. Generally indolent and non-progressive—even regress spontaneously *Diffuse*—spine, innominate bones, ribs and skull generally affected. Mixed pattern of osteoporosis and osteosclerosis. Circumscribed lytic and sclerotic lesions may be present. Diffuse involvement generally in more severe types of disorder	Radiological appearance may simulate myeloid metaplasia, osteoblastic metastasis and, on occasion, generalised osteoporosis of different causes
Hodgkin's disease, 798	345678	Red marrow areas. Bone changes shown in 25% but more common at autopsy	Lymphadenopathy, splenomegaly and other organ involvement. Bone pain later stages	Characteristically, Reed-Sternberg cells (large multilobular with prominent nuclei), eosinophils, fibroblasts, haemorrhage and necrosis. Cellular structure varies from highly anaplastic to considerable fibrosis. Cortex and spongiosa involved as in all lymphomas. New bone—non-tumourous—may be present	Lesions may be osteolytic (commonly), osteoblastic or mixed. May occur without lymphadenopathy so that chest film appears normal. Anterior erosion of vertebral body or increased density suspicious. Adjacent rib erosion almost pathognomonic. Discs generally escape involvement. Para-spinal soft tissue masses common. Osteolytic lesions may cause vertebral collapse. Ribs and sternum often affected. Endosteal cortical erosion and expansion	Course usually 2–3 years but some survive as long as 15. Skeletal lesions frequently respond well to radiotherapy. Marked improvement in prognosis in recent years with newer therapeutic measures. Primary skeletal focus may antedate systemic disorder.

Lymphosarcoma, 798	*456*	Red marrow areas	Short, malignant course, many terminating in leukaemia	Lymphoblasts (more primitive than lymphocytes) constitute bulk of tumour tissue. New bone may form. When lymphatic leukaemia supervenes terminally lymphoid infiltration disseminates through red marrow structures. Difficult on occasion to differentiate histologically Hodgkin's, lymphosarcoma, reticulum cell sarcoma	Mainly osteolytic lesions with diffuse and irregular margins. Grow rapidly, eroding endosteal side of cortex. If multiple lesions, all tend to be of same osteolytic type, whereas in Hodgkin's disease all types may be present simultaneously. Permeating pattern like round cell lesions in long bones.	Transition to leukaemia supports belief that these diseases are variations of a primary disorder of the mesenchymal stem cells
Reticulum cell sarcoma (lymphoma type), 798	**3456**	Red marrow areas. Approximately 10-25% of cases involved	Clinical history that of any of the lymphomas	Although firm whitish-grey lesions occur, tend to be softer than carcinomatous masses. Composed of sheets of cells containing fairly large single spheroid nuclei with nucleoli sometimes present. Mitotic figures common. Intercellular stroma varies in amount and demonstration reticulum fibres by special stain diagnostic. Reactive non-neoplastic bone may be present	Generally osteolytic with mottled permeating destructive pattern although mixed lesions not uncommon. Frequently indistinguishable from other lymphomas	Skeletal involvement occurs generally quite late in disease. Radiotherapy of value
Primary reticulum cell sarcoma of bone, 804	**345**	Major long bones, femur, tibia, humerus, flat bones—innominate bone, scapula, spine and ribs. Approximately one-third around knee	Localised bone pain and swelling. Pathological fracture common, particularly in spine with neurological deficit and paraplegia. Constitutional signs and symptoms generally less pronounced than in Ewing's tumour	Virtually indistinguishable histologically from reticulum cell sarcoma (lymphoma type). Represents round cell neoplasm	Characteristically destructive with permeating, mottled, patchy areas, with wide zone of transition. Findings typical of round cell malignant neoplasm which may simulate Ewing's tumour, although periosteal reaction less prominent than in Ewing's. Soft tissue mass not as large as in Ewing's. Reactive new bone may be present. In spine, collapse of vertebral body with paraspinal mass and block on myelography	Frequently difficult to distinguish from Ewing's tumour radiologically and pathologically in 2nd and 3rd decades. Relatively good prognosis, since response to radiotherapy usually good

TABLE VI. *Diseases of the Haemopoietic System and Marrow* (contd.)
(including Reticuloendothelial Storage Disorders)

B. DISEASES PRIMARILY INVOLVING WHITE BLOOD CELLS (contd.)

Pathological Condition	Age in Decades	Sites of Predilection	Clinical Features	Pathological Findings	Radiological Features	Remarks
Kaposi's sarcoma, 1108	**456**	Skeletal involvement mainly in extremities and particularly lower limbs. Hands and feet not infrequently involved	Four clinical types: *Nodular type*—painful, purplish nodula develop in skin of limbs. Bone involvement unusual and spontaneous remission may occur. *Florid variety*—accounts for half of patients. Fungating lesions of extremities with deep extension and secondary infection. Bone development frequent. *Infiltrative type*—skeletal involvement rare. Invasion of soft tissues. *Juvenile lymphadenopathic variety*—widespread lymph node involvement. Skeletal lesions rare. Poor prognosis	Three patterns described: mixed cell, monocellular (spindle cell), and anaplastic. Fibroblasts and collagen formation occurs during involution. Lesions highly vascular; may simulate haemangiosarcoma or malignant haemangiopericytoma. Considered by some to represent angioblastic reticulosis rather than a sarcoma	Skeletal lesions characteristically observed in extremities, particularly of lower limb bones. Well-demarcated lytic, cortical lesions associated with soft tissue nodules. Medullary expansion with scalloped endosteal erosion frequently noted. Nodules in subcutaneous soft tissues may be demonstrated by soft tissue radiography or xeroradiography. Extensive skeletal osteoporosis may occur due to localised hyperaemia and secondary infection. Widespread destruction of tubular bones of hands and feet may be encountered in advanced stages	Lymphography has demonstrated lymphatic obstruction with abnormal nodes in all cases of extensive disease. Thus, lymphatic system may be initial focus of origin of disorder. Increased incidence in Eastern and Central Europe and Central Africa
Plasmacytoma, 604 This is a precursor to **multiple myeloma (see below), 772**	*5678*	Red marrow areas. Especially vertebral bodies and thoracic cage	Bone pain. Often incidental discovery being asymptomatic until multiple myeloma develops in 2–20 years	Tumour tissue usually extremely cellular with practically no supporting connective tissue stroma. Myeloma cells may resemble ordinary plasma cells with eccentric nuclei—small and uniform in appearance. Such pattern generally seen in *plasmacytoma*	Osteolytic expanding lesions. Especially common in spine, where they are very like osteolytic metastases with collapse. Initially lesions are solitary but diagnosis of 'benign myeloma' is unjustified as they eventually change to myelomatosis. Characteristically no sclerotic margin but can follow radiotherapy. Margins clear-cut. Expansion frequently a major feature	May resemble giant-cell tumour, especially in pelvis, but these tumours usually occur at an earlier age. Expanding lesions similar to solitary metastasis from renal cell or thyroid carcinoma

Multiple myeloma, 772	45678	Red marrow areas primarily, but whole skeleton eventually. Skull often involved, but may be exempt	Bone pain, anaemia, signs of generalised neoplastic disease, pathological fractures	Sternal marrow puncture diagnostic with significant increase in plasma cells. Increased globulin production. Bence-Jones proteinuria 50%. Electrophoretic pattern usually diagnostic—characteristic 'M' spot. In sections from lesion of myelomatosis, cells tend to be larger than in plasmacytoma, with abundant cytoplasm and large centrally placed nuclei. Bizarre, tumour giant cells may be observed in such fields in addition to the small round cells of myeloma	Several patterns: (1) generalised osteoporosis; (2) multiple, small, similarly-sized, radiolucent defects; (3) larger destructive lesions without reactive sclerosis with relatively wide zones of transition; (4) initial presentation as plasmacytoma; (5) sclerosing form Vertebral body collapse common—often associated with large, soft tissue mass and extradural block on myelography. Pathological fractures not infrequent	Sclerotic forms of myelomatosis occur rarely with high incidence of peripheral neuropathy in such cases Relationship to Waldenström's macroglobulinemia exists Amyloid disease may be present in relatively high percentage of patients with myelomatosis and may even precede development of myelomatosis. See chapter on Plasma Cell Dyscrasias, **1823**
Burkitt's lymphoma, 1068	1	Mandible and maxillae. Involvement of other skeletal sites relatively uncommon, with long bones of limbs constituting next most frequent site involved. Lymph nodes, ovaries, liver, adrenal, intestinal tract, pancreas, heart, thyroid, testes and salivary glands may be affected	Most common presentation is tumour involving one or more quadrants of jaw. Other skeletal lesions occur in approximately 10% of cases and may be solitary or multiple	Interesting and varied. Tumour cells have characteristic lymphoblastoid appearance with intense cytoplasmic basophilia and cytoplasmic vacuoles. Uniform, immature lymphoid cells interspersed with large vacuolated histiocytes giving 'starry sky' appearance. Accurate diagnosis requires most critical evaluation of well-handled biopsy material. May resemble Hodgkin's disease or other lymphoma	Presenting jawbone tumour is a purely destructive lesion. Maxilla more commonly affected than mandible. Resorption of lamina dura first radiological sign. Patchy infiltrative process beneath alveolus quickly develops until massively expanding lytic lesion. Radiological changes in remainder of skeleton resemble typical round cell lesions, e.g. reticulum cell sarcoma, Ewing's tumour with diaphyseal predilection. Large soft tissue masses in pelvis and abdomen often due to involvement of ovaries. Renal involvement common and tends to be multicentric with large mass lesions	Exact relationship of Epstein-Barr virus to Burkitt's lymphoma not established. Disorder encountered infrequently in countries outside of Africa, e.g. United States Virtually complete absence of leukemia in course of this disorder in contrast to expected natural history of orthodox lymphoma With exception of choriocarcinoma is only human tumour curable in high proportion of cases by chemotherapy (cytotoxic drugs). Radiotherapy rarely effective
Primary macroglobulinemia of Waldenström, 1118	67	Haemopoietic skeleton, endothelial system, G.I. tract, cardiovascular and central nervous system and kidneys	May be asymptomatic, but usually symptoms and signs of malignancy. Hepatosplenomegaly, lymphadenopathy, bleeding diathesis common. Normocytic, normochromic anaemia. Elevated ESR	Suggest plasma cell dyscrasia with lymphomatous overtone. Lymphocytoid and plasmacytoid cells observed in all areas involved. Increase IgM (macroglobulin) component and beta or gamma spike on electrophoresis	Varied skeletal findings—widespread osteopenia, and marrow replacement pattern may simulate myeloma. Other systems: hepatosplenomegaly, pleural effusion and pulmonary infiltrates, heart failure, thickening mucosal folds of G.I. tract with granular appearance mucosa. Intracranial, subarachnoid and subdural haemorrhages, poor renal function on IVP	Plasma cell dyscrasias constitute wide spectrum of which this entity is one. See chapter on Plasma Cell Dyscrasias, **1823**

TABLE VI. *Diseases of the Haemopoietic System and Marrow* (*contd.*)
(including Reticuloendothelial Storage Disorders)

C. RETICULO-ENDOTHELIAL STORAGE DISORDERS

Pathological Condition	Age in Decades	Sites of Predilection	Clinical Features	Pathological Findings	Radiological Features	Remarks
Lipoid granulomata Gaucher's disease, 764	2 3 4 5 6 7	Lesions tend to be peripheral rather than central. Skull, hands, feet usually exempt. Long bones in adults	Splenomegaly and cutaneous pigmentation. Weakness and fatigue. Acute form in infancy rarely produces X-ray skeletal changes	True lipid histiocytosis. Kerasin found in large reticuloendothelial cells—Gaucher's cells ('foam' cells), deposited in spongiosa, haemopoietic skeleton, liver, spleen and other organs. Bone changes produced in 3 ways; absorption trabeculae adjacent to Gaucher's cells causes osteoporosis, bone destruction by Gaucher's cells, bone infarcts produced by vascular compromise, mainly femoral and humeral heads	Widespread and irregular medullary porosis due to diffuse marrow infiltration. Progresses to destructive lesions with sharply defined borders and endosteal erosions. Abnormal modelling in long bones, e.g. flask-shaped femora. Infarction common especially in humeral and femoral heads. In child may simulate Perthes' disease. Pathological fractures commonest in spine often without clear involvement	Reticulo-endothelial cells enlarge and contain a lipoprotein, kerasin. Appear as 'foam cells' histologically. Particularly affects Jews especially young, but not confined to this race. Pulmonary infiltrations, rare, but do occur. Probably due to enzymatic disorder—deficiency of glucocerebrosidase which serves as catalyst in cleavage of glucose molecules. Results in accumulation of glucocerebrosides in various tissues and organs
Niemann-Pick disease, 768	1	Bone marrow, liver and spleen mainly affected	Infant or young child fails to thrive. Lymph node enlargement, hepatosplenomegaly, anaemia, macular degeneration and blindness, neurological and mental disturbances, and, rarely, xanthomatous skin lesions noted. Death common by age of two years, but number of affected children survive into adult life	Basic abnormality consists of cytoplasmic deposition of sphingomyelin in vacuolated foam cells, resembling Gaucher's disease. Vacuolated lymphocytes and monocytes frequently in peripheral blood smear. Effect on bone marrow may be comparable to Gaucher's disease	Skeletal abnormalities less common than in Gaucher's disease but are reminiscent of that disorder. Skeletal lesions may exist more frequently than believed. Widespread osteoporosis, cortical thickening, coarsening of trabecular pattern and widening of medullary cavities. Modelling changes of long bones considerably less common than in Gaucher's. Tubular bones of hands and feet may resemble thalassaemia. Focal lytic areas and even grossly destructive lesions reminiscent of histiocytosis may occur	Bilateral disseminated interstitial infiltration of lungs may be observed

D. DISEASES PRIMARILY INVOLVING THE COAGULATION MECHANISM

Pathological Condition	Age in Decades	Sites of Predilection	Clinical Features	Pathological Findings	Radiological Features	Remarks
Classical haemophilia, Christmas disease, 758	Signs generally in first two years of life	Major joints, especially the knee. Ankles, elbows and shoulders frequently affected. Spine virtually exempt	Generally males affected in classical disorder. Bleeding may occur due to slight trauma. Haemarthrosis. Patient aware of disability from early childhood. Most haemophiliacs develop first haemathrosis before age of two years, frequently without history of trauma	Due to chronic bleeding into joint, usually due to classical haemophilia. Haemophilia B (Christmas disease) and haemophilia C may be responsible due to deficiency of thromboplastin. In joints, synovial haemorrhages may resorb or rupture into joint cavity. Haemosiderin deposits in synovium after repeated bleeds cause villous hypertrophy, fibrosis and adhesions. Cartilage destruction and subchondral bone erosion by haemorrhagic cavities or hyperplastic synovium follow in late stages with reactive sclerosis, disuse atrophy and secondary degenerative joint disease. Subperiosteal and intraosseous bleeding may occur with pseudotumour formation	*Intra-articular* haemorrhage causes irregular articular surfaces with destruction of articular cartilage and epiphyseal enlargement. Considerable osteoporosis usually present, particularly in active stage of bleeding. Deepening and widening of intercondylar notch in distal end of femur due to bleeding around cruciate ligaments. Haemarthrosis distends joint capsule. Increased density may be noted around joint in contrast to ordinary synovial effusions. In hip, obliteration of venous drainage by synovial bleeding may cause necrosis of femoral head. *Intra-osseous* haemorrhage produces juxta-articular cystic lesions. *Subperiosteal* haemorrhage may erode underlying bone to result in large osteolytic lesions with sharply defined margins— the haemophiliac 'pseudotumour'. Such lesions especially common in innominate bone, calcaneus, femur, tibia, humerus, radius, although may present anywhere in the skeleton	Pseudotumours must be distinguished from aggressive, benign tumours and even malignant neoplasms

TABLE VII. *Arthritides and Collagen Disorders*

Disease	Clinical Features	Common Sites	Pathological Features	Radiological Features	Remarks
Rheumatoid arthritis (R.A.), (adult form), 812	Age incidence from 3rd to 7th decades, predominantly females. Vary enormously from extremely mild, even undiagnosed (most common) to completely crippling forms. Evidence of systemic disease frequent in severe forms—fever, malaise, raised e.s.r., subcutaneous nodules over bony prominences and pulmonary lesions in severe form. In average case, moderately painful joint swellings with effusion and limitation of movement, characterised by exacerbations and remissions.	Hands, wrists, feet, knees and hips although no joint immune. Cervical spine frequently affected	Considered to be primarily collagen disorder. Synovial hypertrophy associated with inflammatory granulation tissue (pannus) which invades and destroys articular cartilage and synovial attachments of bone. Subchondral bone atrophy prominent. Fibrous and bony ankylosis advanced cases. Pannus also in synovium of tendon sheaths and bursae. Serological tests important but not infrequently unrewarding. HL-A antigen tests normal.	In *adult* form—in hand, m.p. joints characteristically involved. In early stages involved joint will show symmetrical para-articular soft tissue swelling (synovitis), periosteal reaction on diaphyses of adjacent bones, para-articular erosions (may only be seen in special views, especially in carpus), varying degrees joint space narrowing, irregularity tendon and ligamentous attachments, and juxta-articular osteoporosis. Later stages, evidence of fibrous and bony ankylosis	Untold numbers mild cases, many undiagnosed. Patients symptomatic clinically represent small percentage of total. Females presenting initially in middle life with hip disease—medial migration femoral head and joint space narrowing with absent or minimal osteophyte formation—probably represent late effects of undiagnosed r.a. Cervical spine lesions important; instability may lead to paraplegia and even sudden death
Juvenile rheumatoid disease (Still's disease), 1050	Usually observed within first decade of life approximately one-third before the age of 3 years. Female to male predilection 3 to 1. Chronic, painful swelling of joints. Fever, lymphadenopathy, splenomegaly and evanescent rash of erythema multiforme type. Pericarditis, pleuritis, uveitis may also be present. Subcutaneous rheumatoid nodules infrequently	Unlike classical rheumatoid arthritis, major joints usually first to be involved—knee, ankle, hip and cervical portion of spine. Small joints of hands and feet tend to be affected later	As in adult rheumatoid arthritis, Still's disease is typically a chronic inflammatory process affecting connective tissue synovium. Associated with chronic hyperaemia. Necrosis uncommon. Destruction of articular cartilage caused by pannus invasion of proliferating synovial tissue. Serological studies often unrewarding	Correspond to effects of peri-articular hyperaemia, with soft tissue swelling around joints as initial abnormality. Followed by osteoporosis, with enlargement of growing ossification centres and often premature fusion of epiphyseal plates. Diaphyseal periosteal reaction not uncommon. In later stages, joint spaces narrow with subchondral irregularity as articular cartilage is destroyed. Resembles changes in adult rheumatoid arthritis, with addition of overgrowth of ossification centres and premature epiphyseal fusion. Organised periosteal reaction may result in rectangular tubular bones of hands and feet. Subluxations and dislocation of joints may develop. Joint destruction may be extreme. Growth of long bones may be retarded and result in very slender limb bones	In advanced cases, spontaneous ankylosis with obliteration of intervertebral spaces and fusion of vertebral bodies occurs in cervical spine in some cases with arrest of growth. Disorder often undergoes spontaneous remission with no residual deformity in adult life. Severe disability may result, however, with crippling deformities, joint destruction, ankylosis and contractures
Psoriatic arthritis, 857	More common in males. Symptoms and signs of arthritis similar to rheumatoid arthritis with painful swelling, stiffness of affected joints. Deformities simulating neuropathies late manifestations. Articular lesions most often seen in rela-	Tubular bones of hands and feet and wrists. S.I. joints and spine may be affected	Inflammatory arthritis closely simulating rheumatoid arthritis with similar synovial pannus. Bony articulations similarly affected. Positive rheumatoid factor in serum only present with concurrent rheumatoid disease (occurs in about 20%)	Classically: (1) distal interphalangeal joints involved initially (in contrast to r.a.) with periarticular soft tissue swelling and articular erosions; (2) usually no periarticular decalcification (cf r.a.); (3) proliferative periosteal reaction tubular	Sacro-iliac joints and cervical spine occasionally may show lesions reminiscent of r.a.; in advanced cases may be difficult to distinguish from r.a. In patients with r.a. who develop psoriasis, combined

Disease	Clinical	Sites	Pathology	Radiological	Comments
(continued — psoriatic arthritis)	tionship to areas of considerable skin, particularly nail-bed, involvement			bones first toe frequently observed; (4) metatarso-phalangeal joints tend to suffer more than interphalangeal joints; (5) 'cup and pencil' neuropathic-like lesions common; (6) fibrosis and bony ankylosis more common than in r.a.	radiological features of both entities may be observed. Sacro-iliac joints and lumbar spine may be affected. Syndesmophytes of lumbar spine similar to Reiter's syndrome. Lesions may simulate rheumatoid arthritis, often involving atlanto-axial area
Reiter's syndrome, 832	Essentially males. Classical triad of non-specific urethritis, conjunctivitis and arthritis. Urethritis can be gonococcal. Conjunctivitis only present in one-third of cases. Inflammatory process of small or large bowel may be associated. Skin involvement including keratodermia, lesions of nail beds, aural and mucosal lesions and prostatitis may co-exist. Skin lesions may resemble psoriasis Arthritic symptoms tend to be acute or subacute, although tend to be milder with less frequent chronicity than in rheumatoid arthritis. Frequently, self-limiting course	Interphalangeal and metatarso-phalangeal joints of feet and tarsus most commonly involved. Hands and wrists infrequently affected. Erosions and spurs on attachments of long plantar ligament on calcaneus similar to psoriatic arthritis and rheumatoid arthritis	Histological findings indistinguishable from rheumatoid arthritis and psoriatic arthritis	Several important characteristic features: (1) periosteal reaction on metatarsals and phalanges tend to be more florid than in rheumatoid arthritis; (2) juxta-articular osteoporosis frequently present, but may be less marked than in rheumatoid arthritis; (3) sacro-iliac joint involvement—joint space narrowing, marginal erosions and sclerosis frequent; (4) syndesmophyte formation of lumbar spine similar to psoriatic arthritis; (5) calcaneal erosions and spur formation, similar to rheumatoid arthritis and psoriatic arthritis	Urethritis may be absent and in its stead inflammatory disease of small or large intestine may co-exist. Serious sequelae of rheumatoid arthritis (e.g. pulmonary lesions) not encountered. Lesions of upper cervical spine with instability, etc., may also be observed in Reiter's syndrome. HL–A antigen present in 76% of patients
Ankylosing spondylitis, 872	Young adult males especially affected. Unusual in females. Low back pain and stiffness, mild pyrexia, increased E.S.R. Early sign diminished chest expansion due to costo-vertebral and costo-transverse joint involvement. Variable clinical pattern in large group of patients from mild to severe. Spontaneous arrest frequent	Sacro-iliac joints, lumbar spine (later thoracic and even cervical). *Appendicular skeleton*—hips, shoulder, muscle and tendon attachments, e.g. calcaneus	Mesenchymal disease of unknown cause—may be collagen disorder. Inflammatory spondylitis in small posterior joints of spine, costo-vertebral, costo-transverse, sacro-iliac (lower $\frac{2}{3}$) and other sites of involvement, including appendicular skeleton. Osteitis of lumbar vertebrae—calcification and ossification paraspinal ligaments. Relationship to rheumatoid arthritis obscure. Small percentage of patients will develop features of rheumatoid arthritis. Serological studies for rheumatoid factor in ankylosing spondylitis consistently negative	*Axial:* Subarticular haziness, erosions and subchondral sclerosis costovertebral, costotransverse and posterior joints thoracolumbar spine. Similar changes sacro-iliac joints (lower $\frac{2}{3}$). Ultimately fibrous and then bony fusion may occur. Osteitis of lumbar vertebrae followed by 'squaring' anterior margins vertebral bodies. Calcification and ossification paraspinal soft tissues and then ligaments. 'Bamboo' spine as disease ascends to involve cervical spine *Appendicular:* Hips and shoulders may show changes similar to rheumatoid arthritis. Erosions and irregular new bone formation, due to stress on tendon and muscle attachments—especially on ischial tuberosities, iliac crests, calcaneus	Proliferative changes ('whiskering' or 'fringing') ischial tuberosities, iliac margins, calcaneus may be extensive and frequently symptomatic. Erosions and new bone formation vertebral bodies probably reflecting osteitis may simulate pyogenic osteomyelitis or even tuberculosis HL–A antigen present in 96% of patients

TABLE VII. *Arthritides and Collagen Disorders (contd.)*

Disease	Clinical Features	Common Sites	Pathological Features	Radiological Features	Remarks
Erosive osteo-arthritis, 824	Middle-aged women predominantly affected with both distal and proximal interphalangeal joints of both hands characteristically involved and with recurrent and acute pain. Nodular soft tissue swelling, redness, local heat, tenderness around affected joints. Flexion deformities may develop. Concurrent cervical and occipital pain not unusual	Distal and proximal interphalangeal joints of hands generally affected and characteristically first carpo-metacarpal joint Upper cervical spine also affected	Differ with stage of disorder. In acute inflammatory phase, synovitis present, highly reminiscent of rheumatoid arthritis. In chronic phase, typical features of degenerative joint disease, with partial disintegration of articular cartilage and osteophyte formation, together with remnants of pre-existing synovial inflammatory disease. Giant cell and lymphocytic infiltration, fibrosis, thickening of blood vessel walls and considerable villous hypertrophy in inflammatory stage	Distal interphalangeal joints prominently involved, but ultimately proximal interphalangeal joints and first metacarpo-trapezium joints. Joint space narrowing, subchondral sclerosis and para-articular erosions generally encountered. Subarticular demineralisation not prominent feature except in acute phase. Subluxation in later stage and fibrous and bony ankylosis may occur Radiological changes in cervical spine indistinguishable from those encountered in ordinary spondylosis	Inflammatory synovitis and subarticular erosions separate this entity from ordinary degenerative joint disease. Heberden's and Bouchard nodes, clinical history and course, and consistently negative laboratory findings for rheumatoid arthritis distinguish this process from a purely inflammatory type of arthritis
Other Collagen Disorders **1. Diffuse systemic sclerosis (scleroderma), 863** **2. Dermatomyositis, 862** **3. Disseminated lupus (lupus erythematosus), 812** (These collagen disorders appear to be interrelated)	*Diffuse systemic sclerosis and dermatomyositis.* Varying clinical course from acute fulminating to mild chronic forms (similar in lupus). Clinical features depend on organ systems involved. Skin frequently but not invariably affected. Complaints referable to G.I. tract, chest, cardiovascular system and kidneys common. May have arthralgia and ultimately deformities of terminal phalangeal tufts, particularly in systemic sclerosis *Disseminated lupus.* Skin rash on face. Cardiovascular, pulmonary and renal manifestations common. Arthralgia hands and feet and major peripheral joints frequent and may be presenting complaint	*Systemic Sclerosis.* Hands and feet (terminal phalangeal tufts), soft tissues of limbs, major joints—shoulder, elbow, wrist and hip (periarticular calcification) *Dermatomyositis.* Major peripheral joints (periarticular calcifications), soft tissues of limbs *Disseminated lupus.* Articulations of hands and feet	This group of diseases classified as collagen disorders. *Systemic sclerosis (scleroderma)* and *dermatomyositis*—principal changes involve collagenous fibres—become oedematous and finally atrophic. Form dense, compact collagenous masses in dermis. Inflammatory reaction may be present. Elastic fibres diminished. Epidermis usually atrophic with flattened rete pegs. Small arteries and arterioles develop sclerosis. Calcification may replace altered collagen of dermis and subcutaneous tissues ('*calcinosis*'). Atrophic myositis common in dermatomyositis. Cystic changes in lungs with hyperelastosis. Sclerosis common in G.I. tract *Disseminated lupus.* 4 groups of pathological manifestations: (1) collagen abnormality; (2) lesions of nuclei of tissues of mesenchymal origin; (3) granulomatous reaction; (4) fibrosis. Small vessels and serous membranes conspicuously involved, including joints, with synovitis. Kidneys invariably affected and heart frequently (verrucous vegetations). Finding of L.E. cells in blood (large basophilic inclusions within	*Diffuse systemic sclerosis.* Earliest findings particularly in hands and. less often. in feet. Soft tissue thickening finger-tips, conical pointing and absorption of terminal phalangeal tufts ('auto-amputation'). Relatively little periarticular osteoporosis. Joint spaces tend to remain relatively intact initially, but destruction of articular cartilage occurs in later stages with marked arthropathy, reminiscent of rheumatoid arthritis. Flexion contractions of fingers with subluxations and even dislocations, particularly of metacarpophalangeal joints. Soft tissue calcifications in hands and around major joints such as knee and shoulder. Thickening of periodontal membrane around teeth in later stages of disorder *Dermatomyositis.* Mainly extensive subcutaneous calcification ('*calcinosis universalis*'). Osteoporosis, particularly appendicular skeleton. common *Disseminated lupus.* Changes in articulations of hands and feet reminiscent of rheumatoid arthritis with periarticular swelling, joint space narrowing and even articular erosions. Juxta-	Other radiological features relate to system involved—gastrointestinal, pulmonary, cardiac and renal Increase in susceptibility to development of neoplasms both in scleroderma and dermatomyositis. Possibly also in rheumatoid arthritis and systemic lupus. In latter subluxations of small joints of hands, particularly thumbs, not uncommon Definite link exists between scleroderma, dermatomyositis, disseminated systemic lupus and rheumatoid arthritis

			leucocytes), characteristic but not specific	articular bone atrophy prominent feature. Joint changes tend to occur far less often than in typical rheumatoid arthritis. Necrosis of bone may occur, particularly in femoral head, without steroids. Sclerosis of terminal phalangeal tufts occasionally associated with vascular lesions	
Multicentric reticulohistiocytosis (lipoid dermatoarthritis), 823	Rare disease affecting adults with nodules and plaques in skin and subcutaneous tissues, particularly around joints. Symptoms of arthropathy, mainly of hands. *Main-en-lorgnette* deformities in later stages with telescoping of fingers may occur	Interphalangeal and metacarpophalangeal joints of hands and other major joints may be affected	Abnormal deposition of glyco-lipoproteins in skin and in synovial tissue around joints, with marked, progressive destruction of articular surfaces of affected joints. Masses of lipid-containing histiocytes in synovium on biopsy	Articular erosions, mainly in interphalangeal joints of hands, with occasionally rapid progression to simulate arthritis mutilans in advanced cases. May be confused radiologically with psoriatic arthropathy. Other major joints may be affected	Diagnosis may be confirmed by electrophoretic demonstration of abnormal lipids. May produce very extensive deformities, particularly in fingers and hands
Sarcoidosis, 438	Affects young adults with higher incidence black race. May be asymptomatic even in presence of skeletal lesions. Clinical history usually suggests arthritis	Tubular bones of hands and less frequently feet, but unusual locations may include spine, skull, long bones and nasal bones	Disease of uncertain cause—primarily affects chest (mediastinal lymph nodes and lungs). Skeletal lesions occur in 10% of patients. Histologically, granulomatous (generally but not invariably non-necrotic and non-caseating) lesions consisting of epithelial cells, foreign body giant cells and asteroid bodies. Periphery of lymphocytes and plasma cells. Positive biopsy liver or scalene node frequently. Negative or weakly positive tuberculin skin test (PPD). Positive Kveim test 85%—a test which is not specific but may be related to elevated serum globulins. Reversed a-g ratio blood serum and hypercalcaemia often	Eight types of lesions in hands and feet: (1) well-defined, generally small lytic defects in metaphyses of tubular bones; (2) lace-like, reticulated, destructive pattern involving metaphyses; (3) well-defined, larger radiolucent defects in phalanges, metacarpals and metatarsals simulating enchondromata; (4) neuropathic-like lesions, particularly in phalanges; (5) punctate or diffuse areas of endosteal bone sclerosis; (6) subperiosteal erosions simulating hyperparathyroidism; (7) periosteal reaction; (8) soft tissue nodules. Unusual manifestations in remainder of skeleton include: (1) lesions of long bones usually as well-defined radiolucent defects with sclerotic borders; (2) lytic lesions of vertebral bodies simulating tuberculosis; (3) paraspinal masses with extradural block on myelography; (4) well-defined radiolucent calvarial defects; (5) grossly destructive lesions of nasal and jawbones; and (6) localised and even widespread sclerosis of haematopoietic skeleton	Relationship to tuberculosis not entirely excluded. Hilar adenopathy and typical pulmonary lesions on chest film often provide diagnostic confirmation. May represent end-stage of other infective processes, e.g. fungal disorders, bacterial lesions, etc.

TABLE VII. *Arthritides and Collagen Disorders* (*contd.*)

Disease	Clinical Features	Common Sites	Pathological Features	Radiological Features	Remarks
Gout, 850	M : F = 10 : 1. Age 40+. Symptoms and signs extremely variable. Usually sudden onset involving single joint with hot, very painful swelling. Severe joint deformities late in disease. Urate deposits extend into soft tissues and may even ulcerate skin. Renal colic and obstructive uropathy possible	First toe ('*podagra*'), other joints of feet, hands, wrists, elbows, knees and heels	In *primary* form increased production of uric acid from glycine or renal excretion diminished. Secondary forms occur in blood dyscrasias, chronic renal disease and as effect of certain drugs. Urate deposits, especially in soft tissues with relatively poor blood supply—articular cartilages particularly, but also in synovial tissues and subchondral bone. Articular cartilage destroyed by urates with chronic inflammatory changes	Usually require multiple attacks before radiological changes. Observe characteristically eccentric soft tissue swelling, narrowing joint spaces, peripheral para-articular, discrete erosions. No juxta-articular osteoporosis (cf. rheumatoid arthritis). Amorphous calcification may develop around joints or in areas of bone destruction. Degenerative joint disease superimposed as later manifestation	Sometimes difficult to distinguish, particularly in later crippling forms, from rheumatoid arthritis. Absence of juxta-articular bone atrophy in gout is a significant feature due to relative lack of hyperaemia of synovium in contrast to rheumatoid arthritis. Pseudotumours of bone may simulate neoplasms.
Polyarticular chondrocalcinosis (pseudo-gout), 854	Mainly in middle age with slight female predilection. May simulate gout. Acute pain and swelling particularly of knee characteristic. Intensity, duration and number of painful attacks of affected joint vary. Symptoms acute or chronic; recurrent attacks not uncommon. Symptoms referable to spine may also be present. May be incidental finding Laboratory studies generally normal except elevated E.S.R.	Mainly knees, wrists (radio-ulnar joint), shoulder, hip and fibrocartilage of symphysis pubis. Bursae and tendon sheaths may be involved	Calcium pyrophosphate crystals deposited in joints with secondary inflammation synovium and cartilage. Intracellular crystals engulfed by leukocytes in acute phase. Hyaline and fibrocartilage calcification typical. Articular erosions simulating gout encountered rarely. Calcium pyrophosphate crystals in synovial fluid confirm diagnosis. Serum uric acid normal in contrast to gout	One or more joints show articular hyaline or fibrocartilage calcifications after evidence of acute synovitis in initial attack. Meniscal calcifications in knee common. Calcifications observed major joints. Juxta-articular osteoporosis rare. Vertical, linear calcification fibrocartilage of symphysis pubis virtually diagnostic. Outer fibres annulus fibrosus of lumbar spine and, rarely, cervical spine, may show calcified deposits. Bursae and tendon sheaths may also be affected and even cartilage of ear. Subchondral bone erosions rarely as late manifestation. Stigmata of degenerative joint disease may follow as late complication	Chondrocalcinosis also occurs in haemochromatosis and primary and secondary hyperparathyroidism. Calcification in and around joints may also be observed in hypoparathyroidism, hypothyroidism, ochronosis, disseminated lupus, rheumatoid arthritis and gout, but calcium pyrophosphate deposition may not be encountered in all these entities.
Haemochromatosis, 855	Abnormality of iron metabolism. An idiopathic form may be genetically determined. Also may be acquired in older patients. Generalised arthropathy, mainly of major joints, of varying severity. Pancreatic involvement may cause complicating diabetes. Cirrhosis of liver common.	Liver, pancreas, skin (bronzed diabetes') and periarticular soft tissues.	Deposits of haemosiderin in structures affected. Calcium pyrophosphate usually present in synovial fluid of affected joints.	Mottled areas of increased density may indicate iron deposits in liver and spleen. Affected joints may undergo increasing destruction with symmetrical narrowing. Juxta-articular demineralisation not uncommon. Second and third metacarpophalangeal joints frequently involved. Calcification of hyaline articular cartilage and menisci common feature, thus presenting another example of chondrocalcinosis.	Haemochromatosis may develop also in such conditions as chronic thalassaemia, particularly in individuals following an excessive number of blood transfusions.

TABLE VIII. *Miscellaneous Diseases of Unknown Origin*

(listed in alphabetical order)

Disease	Clinical Features	Common Sites	Pathological Features	Radiological Features	Remarks
Amyloidosis, 779	Depend on site and extent of involvement, e.g., amyloid deposits in heart will cause congestive heart failure. Skeletal involvement frequently results in pain and periarticular soft tissue thickening which may suggest arthritic process	Hands, wrists, shoulders and hips commonly affected	Tendency exists for amyloid to form around capillaries, traversing intermediate or larger blood vessels. Results in vascular obliteration and tissue infarction. Foreign body giant cells common. Calcification and ossification may occur. Marrow-forming structures in skeleton mainly involved. Amyloid deposits also observed in synovial and capsular tissues of joints, ligaments, tendon sheaths and bursae	Skeletal changes include localised and widespread osteoporosis and solitary or multiple, discrete radiolucent defects, most commonly affecting hands, shoulders, hips and ribs. Coarse trabecular pattern phalanges of hands may be reminiscent of sarcoidosis. Pathological fractures may occur. Amyloid deposits in or near joints may mimic arthritic process, with periarticular soft tissue swelling, synovitis, cartilage destruction and paraarticular erosions. Gross subluxations may result	Classification into primary and secondary forms may still be useful although tendency to discount this currently. Amyloid disease may precede development of multiple myeloma and may follow as complication of same disorder (see chapter on Plasma Cell Dyscrasias)
Carpal-tarsal osteolysis, hereditary, 1110	Rare, inherited disorder autosomal dominant. Marfan-like habitus, pes cavus. Begins characteristically with an arthritic episode in early childhood. Inexorable progress, mainly bilateral. Associated with abnormal connective tissue metabolism. Another variety associated with coarse facial features, corneal opacities, probable autosomal recessive inheritance and abnormal retention of acid mucopolysaccharides	Carpus and tarsus	Not determined	Progressive dissolution of carpal and tarsal bones and later adjacent long bones	Disorder bears superficial clinical resemblance to juvenile rheumatoid arthritis, but joint swelling is not prominent and erythrocyte sedimentation rate is normal
Cherubism, 1022	Bulbous swelling of lower jaw; occasionally excessive enlargement of maxillae. Eyes may have 'raised to heaven' attitude. Teeth widely spaced, may be lost prematurely. Expansion of jaw most rapid in first year or two after onset. Disorder may improve steadily from puberty to middle life, with possible reversion to normal	Mandible and maxilla	Typical of fibrous dysplasia	Bulbous expansion of mandible and sometimes maxilla, containing multilocular radiolucent areas with thinning of overlying cortex. Gross abnormalities of dentition often observed. Individual lesions closely resemble classical fibrous dysplasia	Fibrous dysplasia is not hereditary and affects females more frequently than males in contrast to cherubism which is familial in type, transmitted by autosomal dominance and affects males much more commonly than females. Plastic surgical procedures should be delayed until eventual degree of recession is assessed in adult life

TABLE VIII. *Miscellaneous Diseases of Unknown Origin (contd.)*

Disease	Clinical Features	Common Sites	Pathological Features	Radiological Features	Remarks
Ehlers-Danlos syndrome, 865	Rare. Inherited disorder of connective tissue. Elastic and fragile skin. Articular laxity of hands and other areas. Raisin-like swellings known as 'moluscoid pseudotumours'. Orthopaedic, cardiovascular, gastrointestinal and ocular abnormalities often associated. Tendency to bleeding	Mainly extremities	Underlying abnormality unknown, but defect exists in collagen fibres of connective tissue. Pathogenesis may be concerned with deficit in cross-linkage of collagen fibrils	Subcutaneous, calcified nodules, abnormal joints (hypermobility, subluxation, dislocations) scoliosis and kyphosis and various thoracic anomalies. Skeletal abnormalities include long ulnar styloid processes, radio-ulnar synostosis, short proximal phalanx of fifth finger, delayed ossification of cranial bones, ectopic malformation, and acro-osteolysis Abnormalities of gastrointestinal tract, cardiovascular system, respiratory system, genitourinary tract and dental abnormalities also associated	First metacarpo-phalangeal joints commonly affected with secondary degenerative joint disease. Mild forms of syndrome exist. In severely affected forms clinical stigmata are completely diagnostic. Greatest confusion lies with *cutis laxa* in which joints not involved and musculoskeletal abnormalities do not occur
Fibrous dysplasia, 890	Occurs mainly first 2 decades—3-15 years, but isolated lesions may be observed first at any age. Varying degree of involvement. 1. *Monostotic*—most common form. Often found incidentally or through pathological fracture, with relatively minor deformities, especially in pelvis and femur 2. *Polyostotic* type unusual. Widespread distribution, multiple deformities, bone pain 3. *Albright's syndrome* (associated with cutaneous pigmentation and sexual precocity) rare	Pelvis, major long bones, skull, jaw bones and thorax	Fibro-osseous aberration characterised by replacement of medullary bone by fibrous tissue and new bone. Either fibrous or bony component may be predominant. Fibrous tissue composed of spindle cells in whorled arrangement. Bony trabeculae thick and irregular. Multinucleated giant cells and 'foam' cells may accompany cysts. Areas of cartilage, sometimes calcified, encountered. No distinctive laboratory findings	Solitary or multiple lesions reflecting pathological changes. May have phase of lytic lesions simulating cysts, with thinned cortices, expanded spongiosa and 'ground glass' appearance. In bone-forming phase new bone laid down in medullary cavities with relatively unaffected cortices. Both phases may co-exist. Multiple lesions generally bilateral with tendency to asymmetrical involvement. Disparity in length of limb bones may occur. Children affected undergo early maturation, but with ultimate dwarfing. Progression usually but not invariably ceases when ossification centres fuse	Special features in specific areas include frequency of proximal femur involvement with 'shepherd's crook' deformity; pelvic and rib involvement common with cystic lesions predominating; skull lesions frequent—usually bone-forming—may cause '*leontiasis ossea* variant; mandible commonly affected with cyst-like lesions; sclerotic lesions in maxilla often; spinal lesions rare—mainly lytic. Sarcomatous degeneration unusual complication but occurs
Fibrous histiocytoma—malignant, 1472	Affects young to very old but commonest in middle age. May be asymptomatic. Initial complaint usually painful soft tissue mass of long duration	Thighs, buttocks and chest wall. May be extraosseous, intraosseous or both. Intraosseous lesions often accompanied by soft tissue masses	Several histological types: malignant fibrous histiocytoma, malignant histiocytoma, malignant fibrous xanthoma and malignant giant cell type. All four may co-exist. Varying cell patterns observed in individual lesions but typical tumour characterised by whorls of spindle cells (resembling fibroblasts) with storiform pattern, spheroid pleomorphic cells with multiple nuclei, excessive mitosis and reticulin fibrils. Erythrocytes, haemosiderin and lipids incorporated in cells. Giant cells common	Well-defined soft tissue mass which rarely may contain calcium or bone. Skeletal lesions lytic and grossly expansile. Periosteal reaction may be present. Pathological fractures common	Recurrence after surgical intervention common. Metastases to lymph nodes, lungs and other parts of skeleton frequent and early. Most lesions indisputably malignant. Prognosis generally poor

Gardner's syndrome, 1176	Depend on size and extent osteomata and associated bony excrescences. Abnormalities of dentition. Bleeding from colonic polyps common	Skull, mandible, maxilla, occasionally long bones, ribs and innominate bones. Colon also affected	Osteomata indistinguishable from solitary lesion. Cortical thickening of long bones is non-specific. Adenomatous polyps of colon have typical appearance	Multiple osteomata common in skull, mandible, maxilla. Excrescences and cortical thickening of long bones and occasionally flat bones, ribs and innominate bones. Appearance of colon typical of congenital polyposis on barium enema	Transmitted as autosomal dominant. Carcinoma of colon extremely frequent complication. Other gastrointestinal neoplasms may be associated.
Gorlin's syndrome (basal cell naevus syndrome), 1176	Relatively uncommon hereditary disorder recognised in childhood. Autosomal dominant gene. Many basal cell naevi and other skin lesions present. Cataract formation, corneal opacities and congenital blindness also may be present. Many other anomalies of skeleton, gastrointestinal tract and genitourinary tract encountered. Characteristic facies—ocular hypertelorism and prognathism. Painful cystic swellings of jawbones	Usually mandible—occasionally in maxilla	Skin lesions demonstrate wide spectrum from benign basal cell naevus to aggressive, ulcerating, basal cell carcinoma. Cysts of jawbones are primordial or odontogenic keratocytes—as large as 2 to 3 cm. Typical cysts lined by uniform layer of stratified squamous epithelium covered by thin layer of keratin	Well-defined cystic lesions in jawbones bilaterally. Usually observed in childhood or puberty. May appear before skin lesions. Most commonly associated anomalies of thorax, principally ribs, which may be bifid, synostosed or partially absent. Spinal scoliosis and kyphoscoliosis common. Arachnodactyly, polydactyly and bizarre formation of thumb may occur. Shortening of fourth metacarpal frequent. Calcification or ossification of falx cerebri characteristic feature	*Forme fruste* examples of entity probably not uncommon. Increased incidence of associated neoplasms such as medulloblastoma
Histiocytosis, 900; Eosinophil granuloma (E.G.); Hand-Schüller-Christian disease (H.S.C.); Letterer-Siwe disease (L.S.)	E.G. Benign form. Children and young adults generally. Localised bone pain and swelling common. Neurological deficit if spine involved. H.S.C. *disease*. More widespread, chronic in nature. Children and young adults. Diabetes insipidus and exophthalmos may occur but uncommonly. Lymph nodes, liver and spleen enlargement may be observed. L.S. *disease*. Infants under 2 years. Fulminating variant with fever, skin rash—symptoms and signs of sepsis. Often fatal. Steroid therapy of value	E.G. Pelvis, ribs, spine, skull, major long bones. H.S.C. similar to above. L.S. Skull, ribs, major long bones	Must be considered as definite complex with different but inter-related radiological and pathological sub-entities—eosinophilic granuloma (E.G.), Hand-Schüller-Christian disease (H.S.C.) and Letterer-Siwe disease (L.S.). Depending on sub-entity histological findings vary, with sections containing in varying degrees eosinophils, plasma cells, lymphocytes, histiocytes filled with granules and lipid, fibroblasts, collagen, giant cells and necrosis. Infective cause has been postulated although recently suggested that L.S. disease is form of leukaemia. No distinctive laboratory findings	E.G. Solitary lesions exist in only half the cases with tendency for two or more lesions to appear. Circumscribed lytic defects in flat bones with bevelled edges. 'Vertebra plana' in spine—collapsed vertebral body. Periosteal reaction around long bones with lytic lesion confined to medulla. Lesions may contain small sequestrum. May simulate infection or neoplasm. H.S.C. Multiple skeletal lesions each of which has appearance similar to above. 'Geographic' pattern in skull. 'Floating teeth' with jaw bone lesions. New bone formation rare. L.S. Skeletal involvement in almost half the cases before death. Multiple small lytic defects the rule, sometimes confluent, especially affecting metaphyses of long bones	Pulmonary lesions relatively infrequent in E.G. Fairly common in H.S.C. and L.S. with diffuse interstitial reticulonodular infiltrate increasing prognostic severity. Not a disease of lipid metabolism—lipid deposited secondarily, in contrast to Gaucher's disease

TABLE VIII. *Miscellaneous Diseases of Unknown Origin (contd.)*

Disease	Clinical Features	Common Sites	Pathological Features	Radiological Features	Remarks
Hypertrophic osteoarthropathy, 917	Soft tissue thickening (clubbing) fingers (mainly) and feet. Painful swelling and increased warmth affected area. Limbs may be similarly involved with severe pain and tenderness particularly over tibia. Symptoms may suggest acute arthritis. Associated features of underlying disorder	Tibia, fibula, radius, ulna, metacarpals, metatarsals. Middle and proximal phalanges of hands and feet. Clavicles occasionally	Soft tissue thickening—hyperaemia and oedema. Periosteal new bone overgrowth associated with round cell infiltration may be extensive. Multiple layers of bone due to periodic exacerbations. Cause unknown. ?increased peripheral blood flow due to reflex peripheral vasodilation induced by neural impulses. Seen with *Thoracic lesions*—lung cancer, lymphoma, abscess, bronchiectasis, mesothelioma *Extra-thoracic*—ulcerative colitis, cirrhosis of liver, Whipple's disease, T.B. and lymphoma of bowel, Schminke tumour of nasopharynx, r.a., cystic fibrosis	Diffuse, widespread, frequently symmetrical periosteal reaction mainly confined to diaphyses of long bones and tubular bones of hands and feet (except distal phalanges). Cortex may be thickened and irregular, particularly of tibia and femur. Juxta-articular osteoporosis, particularly of hands, is common	Radiological demonstration of this entity may be initial presenting evidence of underlying neoplasm—usually lung cancer. Periosteal new bone may regress quickly and disappear upon removal of instigating cause, e.g. lung cancer nodule, or even with exploratory surgery alone. *Pachydermoperiostitis* may be an associated variant with no underlying cause, 920
Idiopathic hypercalcaemia of infancy, 1196	Infant 'fails to thrive'. Mental retardation may be present. Appearance of infant in severe cases that of 'elf'. Abnormality commonly transient with spontaneous recovery at end of first year of life	Entire skeleton of endochondral origin	No reports available to authors on histological findings in skeleton. Extra-skeletal calcification reported microscopically in kidneys, blood vessels and variety of other sites. Serum calcium and blood urea elevated. Renal acidosis in 20%. Serum vitamin D activity may be markedly increased	Progressive and increasing density in areas of endochondral bone formation, including base of skull. Growing metaphyses mainly affected. Sclerotic rings within vertebrae. Skull sutures may fuse prematurely causing craniostenosis. Abnormalities of modelling of long bones common. Renal calcification frequent	Dense bone may be brittle and path. fractures may occur. Often a self-limiting disorder. ?Due to hypersensitivity to vitamin D
Infantile cortical hyperostosis, 908	Occurs in infants up to six months of age. Clinical triad of hyper-irritability, swelling of soft tissues and palpable hard protuberances over affected bones characteristic. Infant usually irritable, frequently acutely ill with fever. Anaemia commonly present with increased E.S.R. Spontaneous and complete recovery usually within one year, although chronic cases described. Corticosteroids highly effective	Mandible, ribs and clavicle most often involved. Lesions of long bones less common. Any part of skeleton may be affected, although vertebral column, bones of carpus and tarsus, and phalanges appear to be exempt	Grossly thickened periosteum with normal, mature lamellar bone showing numerous mitotic figures with mucous-like oedema. Hyperplasia, collagen fibre and fibrinoid degeneration as well as acute inflammatory reaction described	Multiple bones involved at different times, although condition generally widespread. Periosteal new bone often massive: tends to affect whole length. Cortical outline frequently lost. Medullary spaces appear relatively enlarged. In long bones, diaphyses affected with sparing of epiphyses and metaphyses. Mandible generally, but not invariably involved	Although almost always self-limiting disorder, cases observed where findings persist, with such late sequelae as fusion between paired bones. Becoming extremely uncommon in recent years. May be confused with vitamin A intoxication, scurvy, syphilis and traumatised child syndrome.

Pacchydermo-periostitis, 920	Rare abnormality, generally self-limiting and familial in origin. Occurs mainly in males, becoming apparent at puberty. Marked thickening skin of extremities and face and history of excessive sweating prominent features. Progressive coarsening of facial features. Gross clubbing of fingers and enlargement of ankles and wrists	Similar to hypertrophic osteoarthropathy	Soft tissue thickening. Periosteal reactions suggestive of hypertrophic osteoarthropathy	Significantly more homogenous and more extensive than ordinary hypertrophic osteoarthropathy. Non-tender florid periosteal reaction with cortical thickening may occur. Bones often enlarge due to cortical overgrowth. Associated acro-osteolysis has been observed	Osseous changes may simulate radiological features of acromegaly; it has been designated *acromegaloid osteoarthropathy*
Paget's disease, 880	Affects middle-aged and elderly mainly. Often diagnosed as incidental finding. Skeletal pain, deformity, progressive enlargement of head may occur. Symptoms generally determined by complications e.g. fracture, neurological disturbances with basilar impression, spinal cord compression from vertebral collapse, sarcomatous degeneration	Pelvis, spine, thorax, major long bones and skull. No bone immune	Three phases. (1) *destructive*—characterised by destruction or replacement of normal bone by osteoclasts, fibrous tissue and necrosis with increased vascularity; (2) *bone-forming*—osteoid and new bone formed on the scaffolding of the replaced original bone in 'mosaic' pattern characterised by irregular 'cement' lines attributed to previous osteoclastic activity; (3) *combined*—in which bone replacement and new bone formation occur simultaneously. Cause unknown. Serum alkaline phosphatase may be markedly elevated	Reflect path. changes—three phases. (1) *destructive*—lytic areas skull (osteoporosis circumscripta), pelvis, long bones, spine. (2) *bone-forming*—new bone accretion to cortex with architectural enlargement. (3) *combined*—bone replacement and new bone formation. Complications include path. fractures, protrusio acetabuli, basilar impression, malignant metaplasia	Almost invariably sub-articular involvement. Potential aggressiveness of destructive lesions, presence of stress or increment fractures convex borders tibia and fibula due to osteoid seams (cf. osteomalacia). Remarkable geographical and racial distribution e.g. common in Great Britain, Northern U.S.A., Australasia. Caucasians especially affected
Polyarteritis nodosa, 921	Systemic disorder which may mimic disseminated lupus. Skin lesions common, consisting of shallow ulcers with clear-cut margins and necrotic bases, especially affecting thighs, legs, and flexion aspects of forearms. Pain may be present at sites of osseous abnormality. Clinical features depend on systems involved	Usually bones of lower extremities	Represents chronic, inflammatory condition of arteriolar walls, but all tissue systems may be affected. Cause obscure. Element of chronic vascular insufficiency may be postulated	Periosteal reaction tends to develop around bones closely underlying skin lesions in relation to inflamed joints. Tibia and fibula most commonly affected although similar changes observed in metatarsals, radius, ulna and metacarpals. New bone formation develops slowly—over years rather than months	May be confused with hypertrophic osteoarthropathy or low-grade infection

TABLE VIII. *Miscellaneous Diseases of Unknown Origin (contd.)*

Disease	Clinical Features	Common Sites	Pathological Features	Radiological Features	Remarks
Thyroid acro-pachy, 922	Definite entity in patients who have suffered from thyrotoxicosis and who have been subjected to thyroidectomy, although actual cause unknown. Thickening of extremities, soft tissue swelling, clubbing of fingers and toes, pretibial myxoedema and exophthalmos occur frequently	Usually hands but feet and lower extremities may be affected	Periosteal reaction with peculiar nodular fibrosis. Reactive new bone formation may resemble hypertrophic osteoarthropathy.	Diffuse periosteal reactions of metacarpals and phalanges of hands and, less commonly, corresponding bones of feet. Distal portions of bones of forearm and leg may be similarly involved. Periosteal reaction tends to be florid and spiculated, differing from hypertropic osteoarthropathy. Diffuse soft tissue thickening and multiple soft tissue nodules may be encountered, particularly in lower extremities	History of previous thyroidectomy, possibly many years before, may be overlooked or its significance not appreciated
Tuberous sclerosis, 1038	Classic triad of facial adenoma sebaceum, mental deficiency and convulsions—not all three manifestations commonly present Pigmented skin naevi, café-au-lait spots and fibromatous lesions of skin and nail beds not infrequent	Skeletal lesions usually in skull, hands and feet, long bones, innominate bones, spine and ribs. Other systems involved	Disorder characterised by presence of multiple hamartomata—representing tumour-like formation and well differentiated but disorganised tissue composed histologically of same cellular structures as organ of derivation. Lesions present in retina (phakoma), kidney (angiomyolipoma), heart (rhabdomyoma or rhabdomyosarcoma) and liver and adrenals (hamartoma)	Intracranial calcifications generally paraventricular in location and hyperostotic zones with sclerotic plaques in calvarium commonly present. Skeletal lesions appearing in approximately half the cases extremely varied. Cyst-like lesions particularly in distal ends of terminal tufts and small contour defects in cortex (cortical 'pitting') frequently noted. Osteomatous-like protuberances on cortical surfaces of tubular bones of hands and feet at musculotendinous insertion sites characteristic. Cortical and subendosteal sclerosis may be present. Long bones similarly affected although less frequently. Areas of increased bone density in innominate bones and spine may simulate metastatic disease or mastocytosis	Increased incidence of malignant neoplasms, particularly intracranially (glioblastoma multiforme) Related to other congenital neuro-ectodermatoses including neurofibromatosis, Sturge-Weber disease, Hippel-Landau disease, congenital fibromatosis and lipomatosis of bone *Forme fruste* cases probably frequent

Werner's syndrome, 389	Occurs generally in childhood or adolescence and most commonly in Jewish race. Progressive thickening of skin of hands and feet, loss of muscle mass and subcutaneous tissues, premature greying of hair and alopecia, evidence of premature ageing, cataracts, diabetes, hypogenitalia, impairment of growth and indolent ulcers of lower limbs	Generalised disorder	Premature and extensive arteriosclerosis and scleroderma-like lesions of skin. Variety of associated neoplasms reported	Extensive arterial calcification coronary arteries, aorta and arteries of extremities. Intracardiac calcifications aortic and mitral areas common. Cardiac enlargement and congestive failure. In extremities linear and spheroid calcifications in soft tissues, particularly around bony prominences, soft tissue atrophy of limbs, degenerative joint disease, osteomyelitis, suppurative arthritis, neurotrophic changes of feet resembling diabetes. Premature degenerative disease of spine common feature. Generalised osteoporosis	High incidence of associated neoplasms. Must be distinguished from progeria

LIST OF ENTITIES SUMMARISED IN THE APPENDIX

The page numbers in parentheses refer to the entries in the main text; those following the parentheses refer to the entries in the appendix.